Therapeutic Medications in Athletic Training

SECOND EDITION

Human Kinetics

Written by Michael C. Koester, MD, ATC, FAAP

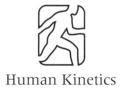

Human Kinetics

Library of Congress Cataloging-in-Publication Data

Therapeutic medications in athletic training. -- 2nd ed.
 p. cm.
 Rev. ed. of: Pharmacology for athletic trainers. 1997.
 Includes bibliographical references and index.
ISBN-13: 978-0-7360-6877-2 (soft cover)
ISBN-10: 0-7360-6877-5 (soft cover)
 1. Pharmacology. 2. Sports medicine. 3. Athletic trainers. I. Pharmacology for
athletic trainers.
 RM300.T52 2007
 617.1'027--dc22

                                                    2007015581

ISBN-10: 0-7360-6877-5
ISBN-13: 978-0-7360-6877-2

This book is a revised edition of *Pharmacology for Athletic Trainers: Therapeutic Modalities,* published in 1997 by Human Kinetics, Inc.

The Web addresses cited in this text were current as of June 2007, unless otherwise noted.

Acquisitions Editor: Melinda Flegel; **Developmental Editor:** Anne Cole; **Managing Editor:** Bethany J. Bentley; **Assistant Editor:** Derek Campbell; **Copyeditor:** Patrick Connolly; **Proofreader:** Kathy Bennett; **Permission Manager:** Carly Breeding; **Graphic Designer:** Nancy Rasmus; **Graphic Artist:** Kathleen Boudreau-Fuoss; **Cover Designer:** Keith Blomberg; **Photographer (cover):** Tom Roberts; **Art Manager:** Kelly Hendren; **Associate Art Manager:** Alan L. Wilborn; **Illustrator:** Alan L. Wilborn; **Printer:** Versa Press

Printed in the United States of America   10   9   8   7   6   5   4   3   2   1

Human Kinetics
Web site: www.HumanKinetics.com

United States: Human Kinetics
P.O. Box 5076, Champaign, IL 61825-5076
800-747-4457
e-mail: humank@hkusa.com

Canada: Human Kinetics
475 Devonshire Road Unit 100, Windsor, ON N8Y 2L5
800-465-7301 (in Canada only)
e-mail: orders@hkcanada.com

Europe: Human Kinetics
107 Bradford Road, Stanningley, Leeds LS28 6AT, United Kingdom
+44 (0) 113 255 5665
e-mail: hk@hkeurope.com

Australia: Human Kinetics
57A Price Avenue, Lower Mitcham, South Australia 5062
08 8372 0999
e-mail: info@hkaustralia.com

New Zealand: Human Kinetics
Division of Sports Distributors NZ Ltd.
P.O. Box 300 226 Albany, North Shore City, Auckland
0064 9 448 1207
e-mail: info@humankinetics.co.nz

CONTENTS

INTRODUCTION

Over the past decade, we have seen an increased emphasis on pharmacology in athletic training education programs and textbooks. This change was long overdue. While athletic trainers cannot prescribe medication, they are often the eyes and ears of the physicians who write those prescriptions. Athletic trainers are in a unique position to monitor an athlete's compliance with medication, its therapeutic effect, and any potential adverse effects.

The use of medications is prevalent at all levels of sport. While illegal performance-enhancing drugs garner a great deal of media and public attention, medications for the treatment of hypertension, allergies, and asthma are used by athletes on a regular basis. Such medications control symptoms and treat disease, allowing athletes to participate in their sport at an optimal level.

At first glance, the science of pharmacology can appear somewhat overwhelming. There are numerous medications with long and confusing names.

Often, the same drug may be commonly referred to by two or more different names! The purpose of this text is to provide a basic overview of pharmacologic principles, followed by a clinically relevant review of the medications that are frequently used by athletes of all ages.

The first two chapters focus on basic pharmacologic principles and the practical aspects of dealing with over-the-counter and prescription medications. The remainder of the text classifies medications based on their therapeutic effect or targeted organ system. Thus you will find discussions of nonsteroidal anti-inflammatory drugs, asthma medications, antibiotics, and antiseizure medications, among others.

Upon completion of this course, you will have a clear understanding of the indications, actions, and potential side effects of hundreds of commonly used medications. This new knowledge will not only foster professional growth but also allow you to better serve the athletes under your care.

CHAPTER 1

Pharmacodynamics and Pharmacokinetics

To be able to advise your athletes regarding medications and other drugs, you must first understand the principles of pharmacology. A drug is a chemical that interacts with and affects living organisms to produce a biological effect. *Pharmacology* is broadly defined as the science of drugs, including their biochemistry, uses, and biological and therapeutic effects.

In the following sections, you will learn about drug action, dosing, potency, drug interactions, and adverse drug reactions.

Basic Principles of Pharmacodynamics

In most instances, for a drug to exert its intended effects in the body, the drug must first bind to a receptor. The receptor, which may be a molecule within a cell or on the cell membrane, reacts with the drug and initiates a biological response that causes the drug to be therapeutic. The relationship between a drug and its receptor is similar to that of a lock and key, so "fit" is critical (see figure 1.1).

Indeed, the slightest change in a drug's chemical structure may completely alter the body's response to the drug. If the receptor is located within or on the surface of a cell, the drug will cause metabolic changes to occur inside the cell. If the receptor is part of a circulating protein, the drug will act by altering the protein's structure, function, or both. Not all drugs bind to receptors in the classic sense, however. For example, instead of binding to a receptor, sodium bicarbonate (an inorganic

KEY TERMS

absorption

add-on interaction

adverse drug reaction (ADR)

bioavailability

distribution

elimination

half-life

hypersensitivity

isomers

lipid solubility

metabolism

peak serum concentration

pediatric dose

pharmacodynamics

pharmacokinetics

pharmacology

potency

receptor

standard dose

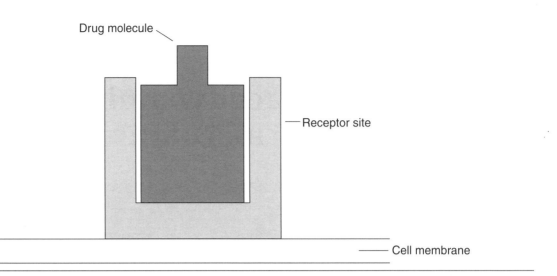

Figure 1.1 The "lock and key" relationship of a drug molecule and receptor site.

Adapted, by permission, from Human Kinetics, 1997, *Pharmacology for athletic trainers: Therapeutic medications* (Champaign, IL: Human Kinetics), 8.

compound) readjusts the body's acid–base balance through a chemical reaction.

Isomers

Most drug molecules have two mirror-image forms, known as *isomers*. The left and right isomers have identical chemical compositions but are arranged differently, much like a left hand and a right hand. As a result, they can have different biological effects. Hundreds of medications contain both isomers, with only one being truly therapeutic. Over the past few years, research has shown that with some medications, using a single-isomer form may improve the efficacy of the medication while reducing unwanted side effects. This explains the recent release of medications such as Xopenex and Clarinex, which are the single-isomer forms of Proventil (albuterol) and Claritin, respectively.

Dosing

Drugs are administered in specific doses, depending on several factors. The amount administered and the frequency of administration may vary based on the specific drug and its potency as well as on the age and condition of the individual for whom the drug is intended. The following are the most common approaches to dosing:

• **Standard dose.** The term *standard dose* suggests that a single-size dose is appropriate for all adult patients regardless of age or body size. Experience has shown, however, that elderly patients may have reduced renal or hepatic function and may require less than the established standard dose. Most orally ingested drugs available without prescription (e.g., ibuprofen or acetaminophen tablets) are labeled with standard dosage instructions. These instructions include the number of tablets to take per dose, how often to take the medication, and the maximum number of tablets an individual should ingest in a 24-hour period. The standard dose represents what researchers consider to be a safe, effective amount of the drug and the dosage frequency that an individual needs in order to benefit from the drug.

• **Pediatric dose.** Nearly all drugs administered to children, as well as some selected drugs for adults, are dosed according to age, weight, body surface area, and the anticipated action of the drug. This is called the *pediatric dose*. At the age of 12, a child generally graduates to standard (adult) doses for most drugs, unless the child is unusually small for his or her age. In these cases, the child may continue to take pediatric doses until the child reaches an average proportionate size and can tolerate standard adult doses. Several formulas are available for calculating the pediatric dose. However, manufacturers of most nonprescription medicines intended for children supply weight and age charts and suggested doses on their product labels to make it easier to determine the correct dose.

Potency

An individual drug's strength, known as *potency*, is perhaps the most important consideration in determining a safe and effective dose. Although many drugs may be available to treat the same condition, some are simply more potent than others. The more potent the drug, the smaller the dose an individual needs to gain the same therapeutic effects. For example, manufacturers typically formulate aspirin, one of the most widely used nonprescription painkillers, in 325 mg tablets. The recommended adult dose for relief of pain and fever is 650 mg (two tablets) every 4 hours. Ibuprofen—a nonsteroidal anti-inflammatory drug (NSAID) that is also used for relief of pain and fever—is more potent than aspirin. Thus, it takes only 400 mg of ibuprofen to achieve the same effects as 650 mg of aspirin. A comparable dose of ketoprofen, the most potent NSAID available without a prescription, is just 12.5 mg every 4 to 6 hours. You should note that just because one drug is more potent than another, this does not necessarily mean that the drug is superior in its effectiveness.

Drug Interactions

Drug interactions occur when one drug alters the effect of another drug. Whenever an individual is ingesting more than one drug at any given time, the potential exists for an interaction to occur. Individual reactions may vary, depending on factors such as the following:

- Genetic makeup
- Kidney and liver function
- The age of the individual taking the drugs
- The presence of an underlying illness or disease
- The amount of the drugs ingested
- The duration of drug therapy
- The time interval between the taking of two or more drugs
- Which drug the individual takes first

Although some drug interactions may be life threatening, most are not. The most common interactions are those that increase a drug's adverse side effects or decrease its therapeutic effects.

Experts generally classify drug interactions in two broad categories:

1. Altered pharmacokinetics: The interaction of two or more drugs alters the way that the body handles a particular drug. For example, phenobarbital accelerates the hepatic (liver) metabolism of acetaminophen; some antibiotics accelerate the hepatic metabolism of oral contraceptives; cimetidine (Tagamet) inhibits the hepatic metabolism of the antiasthma drug theophylline; and some antacids accelerate the renal clearance of aspirin.

2. Altered pharmacodynamics: The interaction of two or more drugs changes the actions of the drugs themselves. This effect can be either inhibitory (each drug decreases the effect of the other) or additive (the similar effects of two drugs add together to produce a stronger total effect).

Add-on interactions occur when an individual takes two drugs of the same type (e.g., two stimulants or two depressants) at the same time. The primary effects of the two drugs add together, creating a total primary effect that is much stronger than what is expected from either drug alone. For example, when a depressant such as alcohol is ingested by a person who is also taking another depressant—such as an antihistamine or an opiate agonist analgesic—each substance compounds the depressant effects of the other on the central nervous system (CNS). The person who ingests two or more depressants may experience excessive drowsiness, dizziness, and a loss of alertness and muscle coordination. In extreme cases, the add-on effects of two or more depressants may slow CNS function to the point of coma and death.

Likewise, combining stimulants such as appetite suppressants or nasal decongestants with caffeine from several servings of coffee or cola may cause excessive CNS stimulation—heart palpitations, tachycardia, insomnia, tremors, and, in extreme cases, a dangerous rise in blood pressure.

Add-on drug interactions often result from a lack of awareness. For example, a person who treats a runny nose with a nonprescription allergy medicine containing an antihistamine and then drinks a couple of cocktails may not even be aware of the risks. Because of the widespread use of so many nonprescription products containing depressants and stimulants, the potential for add-on interactions is quite high and can be extremely dangerous. By federal law, manufacturers must list all active ingredients contained in nonprescription therapeutic medications on product labels and must describe in detail any known precautions related to drug interaction. You should advise your athletes that the best defense against a potential add-on interaction is to study the labels before ingesting any drug and to heed all warnings about drug interactions.

To help your athletes avoid overdose of any specific ingredient, encourage them to pay particular attention to combination products, such as over-the-counter cold and allergy medications. The athletes should know which active ingredients each product contains and should avoid taking any additional medications that contain the same ingredients. Also, remind them to consult a pharmacist if they are unsure of the potential for a drug interaction.

Interactions between two or more prescription drugs can also be dangerous. Fortunately, with the adoption of computerized record-keeping systems, pharmacists are less likely to dispense incompatible drugs to an individual, as long as the individual has all prescriptions filled at the same pharmacy. However, since individuals often receive treatment from more than one health care provider at the same time, the risk of being given prescriptions for incompatible drugs always exists. To reduce this risk for your athletes, you should tell them to refer all prescriptions to the same pharmacy. The pharmacist can then check the athlete's record to determine if any previously prescribed substances might interact with the newly prescribed drug.

Drug interactions are by no means limited to therapeutic medications. Alcohol (ethanol), when combined with certain over-the-counter drugs, can have serious—even life-threatening—effects. In addition to the add-on effects of combining alcohol with other depressants, alcohol combined with aspirin, nonsteroidal anti-inflammatory drugs (NSAIDs), or corticosteroids may cause gastrointestinal bleeding. Furthermore, liver damage may result from combining acetaminophen with chronic or heavy acute alcohol consumption.

The combination of two unrelated drugs that are used to treat entirely different conditions can directly influence the effectiveness of one or both of the drugs. For example, salicylates (such as aspirin) increase the effects of insulin. People with diabetes, who are insulin dependent, may experience a serious drop in their blood glucose level (hypoglycemia) if they ingest aspirin. In addition, some antibiotics, including penicillin and tetracycline, may reduce the effectiveness of oral contraceptives.[4]

Interactions may also occur between drugs and food.[4] For example, dairy products exert a negative effect on tetracycline, an antibiotic used to treat microbial infections. Thus, swallowing tetracycline with milk may interfere with absorption of the medication, potentially limiting its effectiveness. In contrast, certain foods may increase the absorption of a drug. For example, foods high in fat improve the absorption of griseofulvin, an antifungal agent prescribed for the treatment of ringworm infections of the skin, hair, and nails.

Adverse Drug Reactions (ADRs)

Any drug effect that is undesirable is considered to be an adverse drug reaction (ADR). An adverse drug reaction may range from a simple side effect, such as the drowsiness that often accompanies using an antihistamine, to a severe allergic reaction that is brought on by hypersensitivity (abnormal sensitivity that is likely to induce an overreaction to a particular substance). Examples of allergic reactions linked to the ingestion of specific drugs include a rash from ampicillin, bronchospasm from aspirin, and anaphylactic shock from penicillin.

Adverse drug reactions can be classified as either local or systemic. Local drug reactions are limited to a particular site and usually result from topical administration of a substance. In contrast, systemic drug reactions are generalized and affect the entire body. In most cases, adverse drug reactions are immediate (acute). For example, individuals who are hypersensitive to aspirin or NSAIDs will experience acute bronchospasm immediately following administration of either substance. Likewise, an adverse drug reaction to cocaine is marked by acute hypertension or cardiac arrhythmias shortly after ingestion.

Adverse reactions to drugs can also be delayed. Some occur only as the result of chronic (long-term) use. An example of a delayed reaction is the hepatotoxicity that has been linked to long-term overuse of acetaminophen (Tylenol) or anabolic steroids. Another example is osteoporosis that can result from long-term use of systemic corticosteroids.

Adverse reactions may vary significantly from one drug to the next, so it is impossible to generalize about the signs of a drug reaction. However, if ingesting a medication seems to worsen an athlete's symptoms or cause new symptoms, you should assume that this may be the result of an adverse drug reaction and seek medical attention.

Remind athletes that even though a medication is available without a prescription, there is still the risk for potential adverse reactions. Nonprescription drugs, although often less potent than their prescription counterparts, can be quite dangerous if an individual uses them incorrectly or for prolonged periods of time. For example, researchers have found that prolonged use of acetaminophen (Tylenol)—even at recommended doses and without combining with alcohol—causes liver damage. Overusing ibuprofen (Advil) can lead to bleeding or ulcers in the gastrointestinal tract.

Medications During Pregnancy

The possibility of pregnancy must always be considered when administering or prescribing medication to women of child-bearing age. Unfortunately, the safety of many drugs given to pregnant women is uncertain. Medications are rarely tested during pregnancy, so the effects of drugs on mothers and fetuses are typically extrapolated from animal tests or case studies of individual mothers, fetuses, and infants. Only a few medications have been tested in pregnant human subjects and have been shown to be safe. Thus, you should remind athletes who are or may be pregnant to consult a physician or pharmacist before taking a new medication.

Basic Principles of Pharmacokinetics

Pharmacokinetics is the study of how the body handles a drug. As an athletic trainer, you can help monitor this process to ensure that the drug delivers its intended therapeutic effect. Several factors— including genetic makeup, underlying disease, nutrition, environment, concurrent drug therapy, and even exercise—influence an individual's physiological functions and may therefore affect the way that his or her body responds to a particular medication.[4,5] In the following sections, you will learn the distinct components of pharmacokinetics, the routes of drug administration, and specifics about drug concentration.

At its most basic level, pharmacokinetics may be described as a process encompassing four distinct kinetic phases: absorption, distribution, metabolism, and elimination (ADME). All drugs entering the body (except those entering intravenously)

progress through these phases in the following order (see figure 1.2).

Absorption (A)

Before a medication can exert its intended therapeutic effects, it must be absorbed into the bloodstream and circulated through the body. Several factors can influence the speed, rate, and extent of a drug's absorption and consequently affect whether the drug produces a therapeutic effect. These factors include the drug's solubility (its ability to form into a solution in the gastrointestinal tract), the intended site's surface area (skin or gastrointestinal tract), and the specific route of administration.

Routes of Drug Administration

Drugs can be administered in a variety of ways. The route of administration depends on the patient's condition, the specific drug, and whether the drug's desired effect is meant to be local or systemic. Because the majority of drugs pass from mouth to stomach to intestines before reaching the bloodstream, the term *absorption* is generally used to describe absorption from the gastrointestinal (GI) tract into the circulatory system. This term, however, may also refer to assimilation from parenteral injection or topical application.

• **Enteral administration** refers to those routes that involve absorption of a medication by the gastrointestinal system. These include oral, buccal (inside the cheek or on the gum), sublingual (under the tongue), and rectal. Oral (swallowing) is perhaps the most common route of administration for systemic effects. Orally administered drugs are absorbed within the digestive system and pass through the liver before entering the general

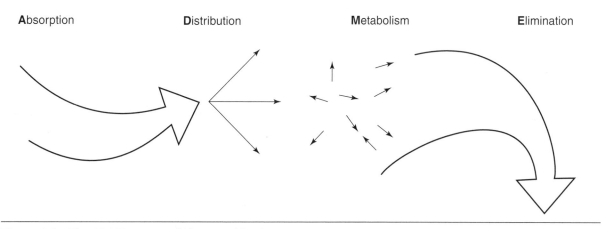

Absorption **Distribution** **Metabolism** **Elimination**

Figure 1.2 The ADME process of pharmacokinetics.

circulation. The liver may metabolize, or break down, drugs and thus can decrease the amount of the drug that reaches the intended site. Buccal and sublingual medications also typically result in systemic effects. Sublingual medications are dissolved in the saliva and absorbed by the superficial vessels in the oral mucosa. Such substances are able to enter the circulation without passing through the liver. Suppositories are inserted into the rectum for either systemic or local effects. Obviously, these agents are absorbed via the lower gastrointestinal tract.

• **Parenteral administration** means that medications are introduced into the body in a manner other than through the digestive system. Intramuscular, subcutaneous, intravenous, and intra-articular injections are typically classified as parenteral.

• **Intranasal and oral inhalation** are other routes of administration designed to produce systemic effects.

• **Topical applications** include drugs administered via the eye (ophthalmic), ear (otic), and skin that generally produce local effects. However, in some cases, drugs administered by these routes may also generate systemic effects if they are absorbed through the skin or mucous membranes.

Effectiveness

You and your athletes should be aware that exercise may decrease the absorption of orally ingested drugs by diverting blood flow to the skeletal muscles and away from the GI tract. Of course, when the body absorbs less of a drug, the drug's effectiveness may decrease.

Patients will feel the most immediate relief from drugs administered by intravenous (IV) injection, by oral or nasal inhalation, or by sublingual absorption. In contrast, orally ingested drugs may take 30 minutes or more to provide relief. Of these, liquid formulations and powders dissolved in water or other liquids before ingestion are faster acting than capsules or tablets, which must dissolve inside the body. Table 1.1 summarizes the various routes for administering medications.

Furthermore, absorption may be influenced by the drug's *bioavailability*. This term refers to the amount of a drug that is actually active in the body tissues and therefore able to exert a therapeutic effect. Orally administered drugs rarely have complete bioavailability. For example, simply taking a 500 mg dose of a medication is no guarantee that 500 mg of that substance will actually enter the bloodstream. Typically, the drug's bioavailability is only a fraction of its dosage size (e.g., for a drug that researchers say is 50% bioavailable, the body will only absorb 250 mg of a 500 mg dose into the bloodstream).

Distribution (D)

Once absorption is complete, the drug is ready for the circulatory system to distribute it throughout the body so that it can exert its intended therapeutic effects. Target sites for distribution are those body compartments and fluids that a drug molecule can most easily seep into. The target site is largely a factor of the drug's function. For example, manufacturers develop some drugs specifically to penetrate the blood-brain barrier and thereby enter the central nervous system; researchers can readily detect these drugs in cerebrospinal

Table 1.1 Routes for Administering Medications

Primary breadth of effects	Route of administration	Site
Systemic	Enteral	Oral Buccal (inside cheek or gum) Sublingual (under tongue) Rectal
	Parenteral (injection)	Intramuscular Subcutaneous Intravenous Intra-articular
	Inhalation	Nasal or oral
Local	Topical	Eye Ear Skin

fluid. Other drugs may more easily penetrate the synovial (joint) fluid.

Exercise seems to have a significant effect on the distribution of most medications. By increasing cardiac output, exercise may increase the speed at which the circulatory system carries drugs entering the bloodstream to their target sites. Additionally, increased levels of catecholamines and other hormones during exercise may influence the distribution, action, and elimination of medications. These increased hormone levels affect the permeability of many cell membranes and alter enzyme kinetics.[3]

The distribution process may also be influenced by the drug's lipid solubility. Drugs that have high lipid solubility can easily penetrate fat stores and cross membrane barriers, including the blood-brain barrier. Unlike water-soluble drugs, which the body can readily eliminate, lipid-soluble drugs may be stored by the body, which means these drugs may have longer-lasting effects.

Metabolism (M)

Metabolism is a clearing process that is the sum of all chemical processes that take place in the body as they relate to the movement of nutrients in the blood, resulting in growth, energy, release of wastes, and other vital body functions. The metabolism of drugs is usually carried out by the liver. In special cases, however, the body may metabolize a drug inside the GI tract or with enzymes in the kidney before the bloodstream can absorb the drug.

Although exercise increases the overall rate of metabolism, which then improves cellular permeability, increased physical activity can actually decrease the clearance of some drugs from the body. For example, during exercise, the circulatory system shunts blood away from the stomach, intestines, and liver in favor of the skeletal muscles. Because the bloodstream delivers less of a drug to the liver during heavy physical activity, the clearance of drugs that are metabolized by the liver may decrease. But since the duration of action for most drugs is usually longer than the activity, the acute effects of exercise on the metabolism of these drugs appear to be insignificant. Still, since physically fit individuals generally experience an increased resting metabolic rate compared to people who are deconditioned, you should be aware that the outcome of drug therapy may be different for athletes than for nonathletes.[1,2]

Elimination (E)

Elimination (excretion) represents the final process whereby the body removes a substance. The body may eliminate drugs from body tissues and organs through the kidneys (urinary-renal excretion), biliary tract (fecal excretion), lungs (respiratory excretion), or sweat glands.

The body excretes the vast majority of drugs through the kidneys. Since blood flow to the kidneys decreases with increased physical activity, the athlete's body may eliminate these drugs at a much slower rate during exercises. You should also remember that very warm temperatures or high humidity can cause fluid loss in athletes who are not properly hydrated. Such conditions can lead to hemoconcentration, elevated heart rate, smaller stroke volume, and increased core temperature, all of which may be detrimental to performance and may affect the action of certain drugs.

The length of time it takes to eliminate a particular drug from the body is an important factor in determining the drug's duration of action. A drug is often categorized according to its half-life, which is the time required for the body to eliminate one-half of a dosage of the substance by regular physical processes. Thus, a drug with a half-life of 8 hours needs 8 hours for the blood concentration to decrease from 10 mcg/ml to 5, another 8 hours to decrease from 5 mcg/ml to 2.5, and so forth. Keep in mind that water-soluble drugs are more readily eliminated from the body and have shorter half-lives than lipid-soluble drugs, which may be stored in the body for long periods of time.

As a general rule, the most intense effects of a drug occur when peak serum concentration—the highest level of the drug in the bloodstream—is attained or shortly thereafter. If you and your athletes are concerned about eligibility requirements for specific events, you need to recognize that tests may potentially detect any drug in the blood or urine long after the serum concentration has peaked. The duration that a drug remains detectable is dependent on its half-life and how it is stored within the body. Substances such as vitamin A can accumulate in fat tissue and be detectable for months after ingestion.

The concentrations of only about 15 to 20 drugs in the blood or urine are routinely measured. Most commonly, serum medication levels are used to track medication levels in athletes with seizure disorders, because the effectiveness of the medication in preventing seizures is directly related to its concentration in the bloodstream. In sports medicine, testing routinely assesses the urine concentrations of many types of drugs, and the results of such tests may influence an athlete's eligibility for competition.

Guidelines for the Athletic Trainer

Pharmacology is a complicated topic that cannot be adequately described in a single chapter. For drug administration and dosing, however, you should remember the following:

- Although an appropriate (safe and effective) dose for a patient usually exists, standard doses do not exist for every drug product. Dosing information as it pertains to a specific drug is provided on the product label. When in doubt about the appropriate dose for a particular athlete or a specific condition, you should consult a physician or pharmacist.

- Most, but not all, drug interactions are undesirable. In some cases, a physician may intentionally use drugs in combination to achieve a desired synergistic effect, but most often, physicians will attempt to avoid interactions. Drug interactions are not limited to prescription medications. You must be alert for the possibility of interaction between *any* two medications, prescription or nonprescription, or between a drug and either alcohol or food.

- Adverse reactions can occur with any drug, even those applied topically. You must know how to recognize the signs of a drug reaction and be prepared to act accordingly. For serious systemic reactions such as anaphylactic shock, you should keep this in mind: The more quickly the adverse reaction occurs following ingestion of a drug, the greater the individual's hypersensitivity to the substance and the more devastating its effects are likely to be.

- Drugs administered by injection and inhalation generally take effect faster than those that are swallowed. Onset of effects after sublingual administration is faster than with oral administration.

- Drug concentrations in the bloodstream may rise and fall in relationship to dosing. In general, drug effects, whether therapeutic or adverse, reach their maximum level when serum concentrations are highest. However, keep in mind that the four kinetic processes (ADME) described earlier in this chapter can affect serum drug concentrations and may, in turn, influence an individual's response to the intended therapy.

- You must be aware of any medications your athletes are taking. Always ask questions before suggesting the use of even a seemingly innocuous substance such as aspirin. To avoid the possibility of an adverse reaction, be specific when inquiring about any drugs your athletes may be taking. This is especially important when working with female athletes who may be taking oral contraceptives, because research shows that the effectiveness of these drugs may be reduced by some antibiotics. Many women don't think of their birth control pills as drugs and may neglect to mention them when asked, "What other drugs do you take?" You should ask your athletes to mention *all* types of pills, nasal sprays, ointments, and so on that they may be using for therapeutic purposes before letting them ingest any additional substances.

References and Resources

1. Boel, J., L.B. Andersen, B. Rasmussen, S.H. Hansen, and M. Dossing. 1984. Hepatic drug metabolism and physical fitness. *Clinical Pharmacology and Therapeutics* July:121-126.

2. Dossing, M. 1985. Effect of acute and chronic exercise on hepatic drug metabolism. *Clinical Pharmacokinetics* 10:426-431.

3. Hargreaves, M., ed. 1995. *Exercise metabolism.* Champaign, IL: Human Kinetics.

4. Harkness, R. 1991. *Drug interactions guide book.* Englewood Cliffs, NJ: Prentice Hall.

5. Mangus, B.C., and M.G. Miller. 2005. *Pharmacology application in athletic training.* Philadelphia: FA Davis.

CHAPTER 2

Practical Issues Regarding Medications

The fact that a product is marketed and packaged in tablet or capsule form does not automatically make it a therapeutic drug. Many nutritional supplements and other products masquerade as "drugs" on store shelves. The term *therapeutic drug* applies only to those substances that research has shown to have healing or curative powers.

Prescription medications can all be considered therapeutic drugs. Street drugs are not considered therapeutic. *Street drugs* is a term used to denote illicit substances—such as LSD, mescaline, heroin, and crack cocaine—that can be purchased for cash on the street. Some therapeutic drugs (e.g., Valium, morphine, codeine, anabolic steroids) can be considered street drugs if users obtain them illegally without a prescription and from sources other than a licensed pharmacy. Experts consider therapeutic drugs sold on the street to be potential drugs of abuse; therefore, the federal government has labeled them as controlled substances. According to the Controlled Substances Act, passed by Congress in 1970, these drugs fall into one of five separate categories (schedules), depending on the likelihood of abuse (see table 2.1).

KEY TERMS

brand name

combination product

comparative negligence

confidentiality

contributory negligence

controlled substances

Food and Drug Administration (FDA)

food supplement

generic name

malpractice

over-the-counter (OTC) drugs

shelf life

single-ingredient product

standard of care

street drugs

therapeutic drugs

Over-the-Counter Medications

Although all prescription drugs can be considered therapeutic, not all therapeutic drugs are available by prescription only. Drugs considered safe for self-administration are available without a prescription. Those over-the-counter (OTC) drugs are therapeutic because they offer treatment for minor illnesses, injuries, and other maladies. The Food and Drug Administration (FDA) must approve both the drug and the information on the label. To be approved for OTC use, a drug must have a low incidence of side effects and low potential for harm *when the patient*

Table 2.1 Controlled Substances[2]

Schedule I	a. The drug or other substance has a high potential for abuse. b. The drug or other substance has no currently accepted medical use in treatment in the United States. c. There is a lack of accepted safety for use of the drug or other substance under medical supervision. *Examples:* heroin, peyote, LSD
Schedule II	a. The drug or other substance has a high potential for abuse. b. The drug or other substance has a currently accepted medical use in treatment in the United States or a currently accepted medical use with severe restrictions. c. Abuse of the drug or other substance may lead to severe psychological or physical dependence. *Examples:* methylphenidate (Ritalin), meperidine (Demerol), oxycodone (Percocet)
Schedule III	a. The drug or other substance has a potential for abuse that is less than the drugs or other substances in schedules I and II. b. The drug or other substance has a currently accepted medical use in treatment in the United States. c. Abuse of the drug or other substance may lead to moderate or low physical dependence or high psychological dependence. *Examples:* codeine, hydrocodone (Vicodin, Lortab), anabolic steroids (including prohormones such as androstenedione and androstenediol)
Schedule IV	a. The drug or other substance has a low potential for abuse relative to the drugs or other substances in schedule III. b. The drug or other substance has a currently accepted medical use in treatment in the United States. c. Abuse of the drug or other substance may lead to limited physical dependence or psychological dependence relative to the drugs or other substances in schedule III. *Examples:* diazepam (Valium), lorazepam (Ativan), propoxyphene (Darvocet), Ambien
Schedule V	a. The drug or other substance has a low potential for abuse relative to the drugs or other substances in schedule IV. b. The drug or other substance has a currently accepted medical use in treatment in the United States. c. Abuse of the drug or other substance may lead to limited physical dependence or psychological dependence relative to the drugs or other substances in schedule IV. *Examples:* diphenoxylate hydrochloride (Lomotil), codeine phosphate (Robitussin AC)

follows the directions for use. Many OTC products can produce severe side effects if the directions are not properly followed.[10]

In the United States, the FDA, an agency of the U.S. Department of Health and Human Services, is responsible for overseeing the manufacture, labeling, and distribution of food, cosmetics, and other chemical substances, including therapeutic drugs. For purposes of monitoring and licensing, the FDA defines a drug as "any articles intended for use in the diagnosis, cure, mitigation, treatment or prevention of disease in man or other animals; and articles (other than food) intended to affect the structure or any function of the body of man or other animals. . . ."[5]

In 1994, the United States Congress approved the Dietary Supplement Health and Education Act (DSHEA). This act allows any company to promote a "natural substance" with claims of improved func-

tion (strength, endurance, and so forth) and health, as long as no claim is made that the supplement actually affects a disease process. According to the DSHEA, for a dietary supplement to be considered a food, it must contain at least one of the following: vitamins, minerals, herbs or botanicals, amino acids, metabolites, or constituents or extracts of any of the previously named substances.[3]

The distinction between drugs and dietary supplements is often a fine one and may depend on advertising claims. For example, if a manufacturer only promotes vitamin C capsules as "being essential to good nutrition," the FDA considers the capsules a food. If, however, the manufacturer promotes the capsules as a cure for the common cold, the capsules are viewed by the FDA as drugs. As such, the capsules are subject to more stringent federal guidelines regarding safety, efficacy, and labeling.

In the United States, all substances that manufacturers label as therapeutic drugs—whether sold by prescription or over the counter—must undergo a series of tests and must meet strict federal standards before manufacturers can make them available to the public. The FDA does not require products that manufacturers classify as dietary supplements to meet the same guidelines as therapeutic drugs. Although drugs are more carefully monitored than vitamins and other nutrients, consumers must still exercise caution in the use of any substance that is designed to alter the function of the human body. Indeed, FDA scrutiny does not necessarily guarantee the safety of such substances.

Generic and Brand-Name Medications

Both prescription and nonprescription drugs are available in generic and brand-name formulations. The generic name of a drug is simply its official assigned name. Drugs are licensed by the FDA under their generic names; however, individual manufacturers may market the same drug under a trademark, or brand name. For example, ibuprofen is the generic name for a particular nonsteroidal anti-inflammatory drug (NSAID) sold over the counter, while brand names for this same drug include Advil and Motrin. Likewise, Valium, available only by prescription, is one manufacturer's brand name for the generic tranquilizer diazepam.

Are brand-name drugs and their generic equivalents the same? In most cases, yes. Acetaminophen labeled simply as "nonaspirin tablets" is chemically identical to the acetaminophen tablets that carry the brand name Tylenol. The major difference is in packaging and price, with brand-name drugs tending to be slightly more expensive. You should teach your athletes that when selecting from several available drugs on store shelves, they should always read and compare the active ingredients listed on the labels. If in doubt about whether products are indeed equivalent, the athletes should consult a physician or pharmacist.

Guidelines for Storing and Dispensing Medications

The administration, storage, and dispensing of both OTC and prescription medications is a com-

plicated and multifaceted process for athletic trainers. Although not often written with the athletic training profession specifically in mind, multiple state and federal laws and regulations apply to the storage and use of medications in the athletic training room. These can sometimes be confusing and cumbersome, but the guiding purpose of all such laws is to maintain safety for the athletes.

Because laws and regulations vary throughout the United States, *you must be aware of the specific rules in your state.* A state-by-state overview is beyond the scope of this text. A recent survey of certified athletic trainers in the collegiate setting found poor compliance with federal drug law, underscoring the need for all athletic trainers to be aware of state and federal laws.[7] At a minimum, you should maintain the following:

1. Medication inventory indicating the following information:
   a. Expiration dates for each medication
   b. Record of each time a medication is dispensed—when and to whom dispensed (must be kept confidential in a locked file)
2. Medication policy book with guidelines for the following procedures:
   a. Dispensing various types of medications
   b. Storing various medications
3. Locked cabinet for storing medication
4. Locked bag for storing medication while traveling

Understanding School Policies About Minors

If you work as an athletic trainer in the high school setting, you must be very cautious about the availability of OTC medications in the athletic training room. Regulations regarding the distribution of common OTC medications, including ibuprofen and acetaminophen, to minors may vary between states and school districts. Unless your school district *specifically approves* your dispensing of OTC medications to student-athletes for certain indications, you should not have such medications available.

Sharing Medications

Prescription medications are dispensed in a specific amount to a specific individual for treatment of a specific condition. It may be tempting for an athlete to pass along a few pills to a teammate, friend, or relative complaining of similar symptoms.

However, the dose prescribed for one individual may not be right for another. In addition, another person might experience an allergic reaction to a prescription medication meant for someone else. Sharing eye drops or ear drops can cause an infection to be transmitted from one person to another via the dropper. Thus, you should teach athletes that sharing prescriptions is not only illegal but also dangerous.

Storing Medications

Most medications, whether in tablet, capsule, liquid, or topical form, can be stored at room temperature. Unfortunately, the most commonly used places to store medications—the bathroom and the locker room—are the worst places, because these areas tend to be continuously damp and humid. You should teach athletes to always check the label for storage instructions. Some medications require refrigeration; if so, the label will specify this. Also caution athletes against leaving ointments, creams, suppositories, eye drops, ear drops, or aerosol canisters in a closed car on a hot, sunny day. The medications may become ineffective because of the extreme heat.

Like most products, drugs have a shelf life, or a period during which they remain effective for treating the condition they were developed to treat. Some liquids lose their effectiveness quickly and may need to be discarded after only 14 days. In contrast, tablets and capsules generally retain potency for 1 to 2 years. If in doubt about the shelf life of a drug, you should ask a pharmacist. Most over-the-counter medications carry an expiration date on the label. For ointments and creams, the expiration date is generally imprinted on the crimped (folded) end of the tube.

Medication Labels

The labels on prescription medications generally contain the following information:

- Patient name and address
- Prescriber name
- Drug name, potency, and quantity
- Pharmacy name, address, and reference number
- Dosage directions
- Number of refills allowed (if any)
- Date the pharmacy filled the prescription

Pharmacists may also add auxiliary labels containing special precautions or instructions (such as "May cause drowsiness," "Take with food," or "Avoid dairy products"). For more specific information about a particular ingredient or possible side effects, you or the athlete should consult a physician or pharmacist.

The FDA requires that labels on OTC medications be more detailed and informative. Consumers with little or no medical background must be able to select the appropriate product and use it wisely without the benefit of a physician's advice. Labels for OTC medications include the following:[9]

- **Active ingredient.** The therapeutic substance in the product and the amount of active ingredient per unit
- **Uses.** Symptoms or diseases the product will treat or prevent
- **Warnings.** When not to use the product; conditions that may require advice from a doctor before taking the product; possible interactions or side effects; when to stop taking the product and when to contact a doctor; a warning for women who are pregnant or breastfeeding to seek guidance from a health care professional; a warning to keep the product out of children's reach
- **Inactive ingredients.** Substances such as colors or flavors
- **Purpose.** The product action or category (such as antihistamine, antacid, or cough suppressant)
- **Directions.** Specific age categories, how much of the product to take, how to take it, and how often and how long to take the product
- **Other information.** How to store the product properly and required information about certain ingredients (such as the amount of calcium, potassium, or sodium the product contains)
- **Expiration date.** If applicable, the date after which you should not use the product
- **Lot or batch code.** Manufacturer information to help identify the product
- **Manufacturer information.** Name and address of manufacturer, packer, or distributor
- **Net quantity.** How much of the product is in each package
- **What to do if an overdose occurs**

Consumers should pay particular attention to the active ingredients in the drug because these ingredients are used by the FDA to assess a drug's safety and effectiveness. Inactive ingredients are those that have no particular medicinal benefits (e.g., the coloring agent or solvent). Single-ingredient products, such as plain aspirin and acetaminophen, contain only one active ingredient. Combination products contain two or more active ingredients; for example, a cough and cold remedy may contain acetaminophen for relieving pain and fever, dextromethorphan for suppressing a cough, and a decongestant (such as pseudoephedrine) for opening nasal passages.

You should teach athletes to discard any medications that no longer have a label. The best way to discard tablets, capsules, or liquids is to flush them down the toilet. Consult a pharmacist before discarding other drug formulations.

Travel Considerations

The best defense against illness or injury is preparation. When traveling with athletes who are minors, you should make sure that any medication an athlete takes is given to you (the athletic trainer) or the coach. The athlete's parent should give you the medication in its original container, along with written permission from the parent and prescription notes from the physician. Athletes who are 18 years of age or older should be responsible for carrying their own medications. When traveling with these athletes, you should be sure that the following items are included on their person or in their carry-on luggage:

- A prescription health insurance card
- Medical history card and allergy or "medic alert" bracelet, if applicable, in case the athlete is rendered unconscious or must undergo general anesthesia
- Enough prescription medication to span the period of time the athlete will be away from home, plus an additional week in case some doses get lost, stolen, or damaged, or in case the return is delayed

Encourage your athletes to obtain refills before leaving home. However, if an athlete's prescription runs out while he or she is traveling within the United States, obtaining a new prescription is often relatively simple. In fact, in many states, it is now legal to fax prescriptions directly to pharmacies. You can ask a local pharmacist to contact either the prescribing physician or the original pharmacy

for a copy of the prescription. It may take time for the pharmacist to reach the prescribing physician, so plan accordingly.

Whether your team is traveling across town or around the world, athletes need to know how to transport and use medication safely. To make every trip go smoothly, you and your athletes should be prepared by having the right packaging, documentation, and other details for all medication. If an unexpected need arises while traveling, you must be prepared to help your athletes get the medication they need as quickly as possible.

Carrying medications from one country to another should not pose a problem or cause extensive questioning from customs officials as long as the drugs are contained securely in their original (labeled) pharmacy bottles. Therefore, instruct your athletes to never carry loose tablets or capsules, place medications in inappropriate containers, or mix different pills in one container. Medications should be kept in the original pharmacy bottle with the label firmly affixed.

It is impossible to address every scenario that could arise when an athlete requires a refill of a prescription medication while traveling in another country. The FDA warns health care professionals and consumers that filling their prescriptions abroad may have adverse health consequences; confusion about brand names for drugs could inadvertently lead consumers to take the wrong medication for their condition. An FDA investigation has found that many foreign medications, although marketed under the same or similar-sounding brand names as those in the United States, contain different active ingredients than the medications in the United States. Taking a different active ingredient may not help, and may even harm, the user.[4] Therefore, the recommended practice is to carry duplicate prescriptions, written and translated for both generic and brand names.[1] This will be especially helpful in the event that medications are stolen or lost.

Travelers should carry sufficient amounts of the medications they may need when traveling internationally. A good rule of thumb is to bring an extra week's supply.[1] All medications should be placed in a carry-on bag and, as mentioned, should be in their original containers with the original labels. Also, you should check with the foreign embassy of the country you are visiting to make sure that any required medications are not considered to be illegal narcotics. If you are carrying a narcotic-based prescription drug (e.g., sedatives, tranquilizers), you should also carry a letter from the athlete's physician to avoid potential problems with customs officials. The letter should state why the athlete needs the drug or drugs in question.[1]

Regulations regarding carry-on items for airline passengers frequently change. Currently, aerosol containers, except those used for personal care or hygiene, are prohibited by the Transportation Security Administration (TSA) in both carry-on and checked baggage. The TSA requests that items such as aerosol antifungal agents be placed in checked baggage. You may bring supplemental personal medical oxygen and other respiratory-related equipment and devices (e.g., nebulizer, respirator, asthma inhaler) through the screening checkpoint once they have been screened.[11] Since regulations are subject to change, you should check the TSA Web site (www.tsa.gov) for updates before any team travel.[11]

Drug Testing

A full discussion of the legal ramifications and scientific details of drug testing in athletics is beyond the scope of this text. The National Collegiate Athletic Association (NCAA) and the International Olympic Committee (IOC) both randomly test athletes for illegal and performance-enhancing drugs. The drug testing and education arm of the IOC is the World Anti-Doping Agency (WADA). Currently, all screening tests are carried out using urine samples only. Several high schools throughout the United States also conduct screening for illegal and performance-enhancing drugs.

You should be vigilant in evaluating your athletes for the use of illegal substances. In addition, you must counsel the athletes on the safe use of "legal" medications that could result in a "positive" drug test. The NCAA and WADA have different regulations regarding the use of several drugs, and these regulations are subject to change. For a complete and updated list of banned substances, you should contact the appropriate governing body at either www.ncaa.org[8] or www.wada-ama.org.[12]

Medical Malpractice and the Law of Negligence

Legal issues may arise from any action taken, or not taken, by an athletic trainer or team physician. This section is not meant to imply that medication use by athletes puts you at greater risk for encountering legal trouble. It is simply included in this chapter to foster further education on a topic that is often not adequately addressed in professional textbooks.

By legal definition, *malpractice* refers to any actions taken that are outside a defined standard of care and that result in harm. The standard of care reflects those rules, actions, or conditions that have been defined to guide the practice of medicine, which investigators can use to evaluate the performance of caregivers. In other words, investigators expect similarly trained individuals to provide the same standard of care under similar circumstances.

For a physician to be successfully sued for medical malpractice, prosecutors must prove the following four elements of negligence:[6]

- Duty: Did the defendant have a duty that was not performed?
- Breach: Was this duty breached?
- Causation: Did the defendant's action (or lack thereof) cause harm?
- Damages: Did the patient suffer actual harm? (Negligence without damages will not result in malpractice action.)

Before deciding whether malpractice has occurred, the court will also take into consideration the concept of contributory negligence. *Contributory negligence* refers to fault on the part of the victim. Did he or she somehow play a part in the harmful action? Could he or she have prevented the harm from occurring? An injured athlete who is found to be contributorily negligent may not be successful in suing a team physician or athletic trainer for negligence or recklessness.[6] For example, an athlete is given specific instructions by the team physician to take three tablets of ibuprofen every 8 hours over the weekend; however, the athlete ignores those instructions and instead takes six tablets every 4 hours. The athlete then develops acute renal failure. If a lawsuit were to result, the court may find the athlete to be contributorily negligent because he ignored the specific instructions that he was given.

In the past, plaintiffs found to be contributorily negligent could not recover any damages, because the system provided for all or nothing. This approach, however, has since been found to be an unforgiving one. As a result, for malpractice recovery, responsibility is now divided between the defendant and the plaintiff.[6] If, for example, the court finds the team physician to be 80% at fault and finds the athlete who sues for malpractice to be 20% at fault, the athlete will recover only 80% of the damages awarded by the court. The practice of assigning proportionate responsibility is called *comparative negligence.*

What the Athletic Trainer Should Do

You can help avoid litigation by adhering to the following guidelines.[6]

- Recognize and follow regulations. Become familiar with common sport-specific injuries, and know the regulations for treating them as established by athletic governing bodies and other regulatory agencies. Do not, for example, dispense Tylenol with codeine tablets to an injured athlete simply because some are "left over." Remember, this drug is a schedule III controlled substance, and any violation of regulations governing the handling of a controlled substance invites legal action. In addition, since the drug in question is a prescription-only formulation, administering it to any individual other than the one for whom it was originally prescribed violates federal law.

- Plan for managing health-related situations and crises *before* they occur. Know when to seek assistance from another health professional. For example, when an athlete with exercise-induced bronchospasm does not respond to his or her metered-dose inhaler, you should seek medical assistance. Know what to do if an athlete is injured or becomes ill in the training room or on the playing field. Have an organizational plan in place that includes the following:

  - Names and locations of appropriately trained personnel to assist in providing on-site emergency medical care

  - Provisions for adequate on-site emergency equipment and supplies

  - Provisions for emergency transportation with appropriately trained personnel on-site or available on call

  - Communication mechanisms to summon emergency transportation and personnel

  - Knowledge of the location of the nearest hospital facility with the appropriate personnel and equipment to handle the situation

  - Familiarity with consultation services that may be helpful in emergency situations

- Always follow the first rule of medicine: Do no harm. This rule applies to the administering of *all* medications. Do not give out over-the-counter drugs indiscriminately. As previously stated, even these widely available medications can cause serious adverse reactions in some individuals.

- Know your job description and what your employment contract indicates is expected of you.

Your employment contract should identify your job duties and responsibilities. Become familiar with the specifics of your contract, and do not attempt to perform duties that are above and beyond your level of expertise or what your employer expects of you. Know when and where to obtain necessary assistance. Each state has separate statutes regarding contracts. So before signing any contract, you should seek advice from an attorney who is familiar with the law of the state as it applies to sports medicine.

- Respect the confidential nature of medical information. Confidentiality is the respect you assign to the privacy of personal information provided to you by the athletes under your care. Like most people, athletes may be sensitive about their medical histories. For example, an individual may not want others to know that he or she has a chronic condition, such as diabetes or epilepsy. *Always* take care to respect the athlete's desire for privacy. An athlete may consider failure to do so a breach of confidentiality and possible grounds for legal action.

Sometimes a fine line exists between one person's need for confidentiality and another's need to know. In her book *Law and the Team Physician,* Elizabeth M. Gallup, MD, JD, notes that the team physician does *not* have a duty to report an athlete who voluntarily discloses drug or alcohol use.[6] Such situations can, however, be open to interpretation. Athletes will not seek help or advice from an athletic trainer whom they cannot trust to keep their confidence. But in some instances, the public duty to *warn* third parties of impending harm may override the private duty of confidentiality.[6]

For example, anabolic steroids are known to cause personality changes and heighten aggressiveness; they may even cause otherwise law-abiding and psychiatrically asymptomatic individuals to develop manic and psychotic symptoms culminating in violent crimes. You must therefore weigh the benefits of reporting to the proper authorities any athlete who appears to be developing these tendencies—or who makes actual threats to another individual—against the potential harm that may result by remaining silent. In such cases, safety must take precedence over confidentiality.

How the Athletic Trainer Can Prevent Legal Action

You can generally perform your job without fear of legal action by observing the four Cs:[6]

1. Compassion. If you have good relationships with your athletes, you are less likely to be

sued than if you don't. Experience has shown that patients find it difficult to sue a physician they like and one they believe cares about them. The same principle applies to athletes and athletic trainers. Keep in mind that in our society, people reward humility and punish rudeness and arrogance.

2. Communication. Informed consent is the cornerstone of good communication between you and your athletes. If an athlete demands to participate in an activity despite medical advice to the contrary, you and the team physician must effectively communicate the risks of such behavior. You must also ensure that the appropriate paperwork—the exculpatory waiver—is executed.

3. Competence. One of the best ways to avoid liability is to maintain clinical competence. So keep your skills current and sharp.

4. Charting. The written medical record is the physician's strongest tool in a court of law. Although charting is probably more of a concern for the team physician than for you as the athletic trainer, you should carefully document all actions, especially those involving therapeutic medications or other types of treatment. No firm rules exist for charting, but common sense dictates that you should describe on paper or in a computer database any action pertaining to medical matters. This may include the dispensing of an NSAID to relieve an athlete's headache or the application of an antifungal agent to cure his athlete's foot. Then you should make such data an integral part of the individual's permanent athletic record.

Guidelines for the Athletic Trainer

Always remember that using medications, whether dispensed by prescription or sold over the counter, is serious business. Even nonprescription drugs can be fatal if someone takes them in excessive doses or turns out to be allergic to the medication.

Know which substances are banned by governing bodies. Also be aware that any combination product that an athlete might innocently consume could test positive as a banned substance because of a particular ingredient. Even simple OTC cough and cold remedies sometimes contain sympathomimetics (drugs that influence the involuntary actions of the nervous system, such as regulation of heart rate and blood pressure). Athletes who test positive for these substances may be disqualified from competition. You should be especially wary of any supplements claiming performance enhancement, because they may contain banned substances.

Advise athletes to never leave medications or syringes lying around the locker room or the hotel room, particularly in foreign countries. For example, if an athlete injects insulin to control his or her diabetes, a hotel maid may find the athlete's used syringe, wrongly suspect illicit drug use, and call the police.

Discourage athletes from sharing medications, even if they are prescribed the same drug. A medication's dose or potency may be entirely different for different people. Make sure that athletes understand that sharing prescription medications is not only prohibited by federal law but is also dangerous.

Teach athletes that despite the widespread availability of OTC drugs and products purchased at health food stores and nutrition centers, these products are not totally without side effects. Nutritional supplements are not subject to strict FDA review, and labeling is not standardized. Although the recommended dosage for most OTC drugs is clearly stated on the label, this is not necessarily true for nutritional supplements.

Be sure to have a medical kit on hand that contains one or more nonprescription painkillers, a topical pain reliever, antiseptics, antibiotic ointment, and antifungal agents. The kit should not be accessible to athletes without the knowledge and approval of the athletic trainer or team physician. When at home, keep all medical supplies in a locked drawer or cabinet. Likewise, when traveling, keep medications in a locked box or bag that is not accessible to athletes without your knowledge.

Regarding the use of therapeutic medications, you have two important roles as an athletic trainer:

1. *As a health advisor about medication use.* As an athletic trainer, you should recognize your limitations with regard to what you know about medical conditions, management of injuries and disease, and the use of medications. Although you may not be trained to answer all health-related questions, your athletes will often assume that you can, and they will turn to you for medical advice. You *must* be able to recognize situations beyond your level of expertise so you can refer athletes to another health professional. As long as you are prudent in following this principle, you should not be afraid to offer guidance on simple medical matters.

For specific medications, you should always follow directions on labels. Likewise, encourage your athletes to take prescription medications as directed and to not exceed the recommended doses of either prescription or nonprescription drugs. Remind people with asthma, diabetes, and other chronic conditions to never skip scheduled doses of their medications because exercise can adversely affect the management of many illnesses. In general, it is always best to discourage combining alcohol with *any* medication, although for some medications, the combination is unlikely to cause drastic complications. Whenever administering any new medication to an athlete, be sure to ask about drug allergies and other medications he or she may already be taking. Always keep in mind that the intended therapeutic effects of one drug may be increased or decreased in combination with another. Moreover, the chance for add-on effects always exists when an individual uses two or more drugs of the same type in combination.

2. *As a watchdog for inappropriate drug use.* In your role as an athletic trainer, if you spot inappropriate drug use, you must first decide how involved you want to be. Ideally, you would do everything possible to both curb and report illicit drug use. If you have the best interests of your athletes in mind, you will discourage the abuse of performance-enhancing drugs so that this problem never develops in the first place. However, you must be aware that despite your best efforts, some athletes may turn to performance-enhancing drugs and then use additional drugs to mask detection of these substances or to counteract their side effects.

Furthermore, tests cannot detect all drugs. For example, injections of artificial testosterone, erythropoietin, and human growth hormone are identical to their endogenous (naturally occurring) counterparts. You should be aware of the side effects of these drugs and keep a drug reference book handy for additional information on such matters. In addition, some drugs are banned in one dosage form (albuterol tablets are banned) but not in others (albuterol inhalers are permitted). As an athletic trainer, you must be able to advise athletes on this issue when competition is near or suggest sources they can consult for such information. When advising athletes about banned substances, do not overlook herbal remedies, which are widely available in health food stores.

References and Resources

1. AmericanHospitals.com. *Common questions.* Retrieved December 5, 2006, from American Hospitals Web site: www.americanhospitals.com/questions/travel/travwmeds.htm.

2. U.S. Department of Justice. *Department of Justice. Code of Federal Regulations. Section 1308. Schedules of Controlled Substances.* Retrieved December 5, 2006, from U.S. Department of Justice Drug Enforcement Administration Office of Diversion Control Web site: www.deadiversion.usdoj.gov/21cfr/cfr/2108cfrt.htm.

3. U.S. Food and Drug Administration. *Dietary Supplement Health and Education Act of 1994.* Retrieved December 5, 2006, from U.S. Food and Drug Administration Web site: www.fda.gov/opacom/laws/dshea.html.

4. U.S. Food and Drug Administration. FDA cautions consumers against filling U.S. prescriptions abroad. Drugs with same or similar names may contain different active ingredients than in U.S. and pose health risks. *FDA News.* Retrieved August 21, 2006, from www.fda.gov/bbs/topics/news/2006/NEW01295.html.

5. U.S. Food and Drug Administration. *Federal Food, Drug, and Cosmetic Act.* Retrieved December 5, 2006, from U.S. Food and Drug Administration Web site: www.fda.gov/opacom/laws/fdcact/fdcact1.htm.

6. Gallup, E.M. 1995. *Law and the team physician.* Champaign, IL: Human Kinetics.

7. Kahanov, L., D. Furst, S. Johnson, and J. Roberts. 2003. Adherence to drug-dispensation and drug-administration laws and guidelines in collegiate athletic training rooms. *J Athl Training* 38:252-258.

8. National Collegiate Athletic Association. NCAA banned drug classes. www1.ncaa.org/membership/ed_outreach/health-safety/drug_testing/banned_drug_classes.pdf. Accessed 10/14/06.

9. *The new over-the-counter medicine label: Take a look.* Retrieved December 6, 2006, from U.S. Food and Drug Administration Center for Drug Evaluation and Research Web site: www.fda.gov/cder/consumerinfo/OTClabel.htm.

10. Mangus, B.C., and M.G. Miller. 2005. *Pharmacology application in athletic training.* Philadelphia: FA Davis.

11. Transportation Security Administration. *Permitted and prohibited items.* Retrieved December 5, 2006, from Transportation Security Administration Web site: www.tsa.gov/travelers/airtravel/prohibited/permitted-prohibited-items.shtm.

12. World Anti-Doping Agency. The world anti-doping code: The 2006 prohibited list. www.wada-ama.org/rtecontent/document/2006_LIST.pdf. Accessed 10/14/06.

CHAPTER 3

Anti-Inflammatory Drugs: Aspirin and the Nonsteroidal Anti-Inflammatory Drugs (NSAIDs)

Prescription and OTC nonsteroidal anti-inflammatory drugs (NSAIDs) are widely used in athletics for both their analgesic and anti-inflammatory properties. In this chapter, you will learn about the origins of these medications, their mechanisms of action, and the proper uses for the medications.

Aspirin

Aspirin is a derivative of salicylic acid and has been widely used as a remedy for pain, fever, and inflammation for over 100 years. Introduced to the American public in 1899, aspirin—or *acetylsalicylic acid* as it is known to pharmacologists—remains one of the world's most widely used over-the-counter remedies for pain. Although aspirin is technically also an NSAID, it is generally not referred to as such. NSAIDs are discussed later in the chapter.

Indications and Uses

In addition to its analgesic (painkilling) effects, aspirin has many uses, as shown in figure 3.1. Aspirin's mechanism of action results from its irreversible binding onto the cyclooxygenase (COX) enzyme, which then inhibits the biosynthesis of prostaglandins.[2] Prostaglandins are hormonelike derivatives of fatty acid that have many functions in healthy bodies. They increase awareness of pain, promote coagulation of the blood, and contribute to the inflammatory process. Aspirin inhibits the production of the pro-inflammatory prostaglandins and thromboxane. Aspirin's effects on the prostaglandins are the reason that the FDA classifies aspirin both as an antipyretic (a drug treatment that lowers fever) and an anti-inflammatory agent.

KEY TERMS

analgesic

anti-inflammatory

antiplatelet

antipyretic

COX-2

delayed-release tablets

NSAID

Aspirin is absorbed very quickly from the gastrointestinal tract—usually within 30 minutes of ingestion. Although elimination is a complex process, the effects of this drug in recommended doses typically last up to 4 hours.

The FDA also classifies aspirin as an antiplatelet—a drug that interferes with the blood's ability to clot. Aspirin does this by preventing the production of thromboxane, a powerful stimulator of blood platelet activation, which is an essential step in the clotting process.[2] Aspirin's anticoagulant effect has both positive and negative implications for users. On the positive side, the blood-thinning effects of a small dose of aspirin taken once a day appear to decrease the risk of a second heart attack or stroke in susceptible individuals.[16] However, when used in combination with certain drugs or used for certain health conditions, aspirin's ability to thin the blood can have a negative impact.

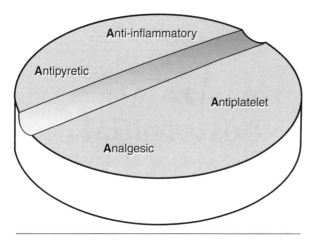

Figure 3.1 The four actions of aspirin.

Reprinted, by permission, from Human Kinetics, 1997, *Pharmacology for athletic trainers: Therapeutic medications* (Champaign, IL: Human Kinetics), 25.

These negative effects are discussed further in the following sections.

Thus, aspirin is an analgesic, antipyretic, anti-inflammatory, and antiplatelet agent. Specifically, in clinical medicine, prescribers routinely use aspirin for relief of mild pain, including headaches and minor musculoskeletal pain (sore joints, muscle stiffness, and so forth); relief of fever; prevention of stroke or a subsequent myocardial infarction (heart attack); and treatment of inflammatory musculo-skeletal conditions such as rheumatoid arthritis and ankylosing spondylitis.

Routes of Administration

Aspirin is almost always administered orally, most often in either tablet or caplet form; chewable tablets and chewing gum aspirin are also available for adults and children who have difficulty swallowing pills. In addition, some users may find enteric-coated tablets (Ecotrin) and aspirin powders easier to ingest. The thin, smooth coating on enteric aspirin briefly retards dissolution, facilitates swallowing, and shields the user from the drug's sometimes bitter taste. Aspirin powders dissolve in fruit juice or water, making them easier to swallow and possibly faster acting than tablets that dissolve inside the body.[16]

Finally, rectal suppositories are available for the administration of aspirin to people who are vomiting, unconscious, or otherwise unable to ingest the drug orally. Rectally administered doses tend to be less effective than ingested doses because absorption of the drug by this route is slow and the suppositories sometimes slip out before the body fully absorbs the aspirin.

General Dose Protocols

Aspirin is generally formulated in 325 mg tablets. For adults, the recommended dose is two tablets (650 mg) every 4 hours, with a 24-hour maximum dose not to exceed 4,000 mg. An initial "loading dose" of 975 mg (three tablets) may be acceptable for faster pain relief.[16] This larger dose should only be administered once; a repeat within 3 to 4 hours may cause an adverse reaction, such as ringing in the ears, which is often the first warning sign of an aspirin overdose. Aspirin users should be aware that drug manufacturers formulate their products in varying strengths. You should encourage athletes to check the label for specific dose amounts and frequency before ingesting any aspirin tablets or caplets.

Unless otherwise directed by a physician, adults should limit their use of aspirin and other salicylates for relief of pain to no more than 10 consecutive days; use of salicylates to control fever should be limited to 3 days. Pain or fever that does not respond to aspirin within these recommended time frames may indicate a more serious condition requiring medical attention.

Side Effects and Adverse Reactions

Although aspirin and other salicylates are effective agents for the relief of pain and fever, you and your athletes should use them cautiously. Adverse reactions to aspirin and other salicylates are well known, and research has documented them extensively. More specifically, aspirin and salicylates may cause some of the following side effects and adverse reactions:

- Gastrointestinal side effects (ulceration, gastritis, GI bleeding, and hepatotoxicity) are possible in anyone who ingests aspirin.[14] The effects are likely caused by a combination of the inhibition of prostaglandin synthesis and the direct effect of aspirin on the lining of the stomach.[8] "Buffered" preparations may lessen GI upset, as can taking aspirin with a meal.

- Aspirin is a powerful antiplatelet, so anyone who ingests the drug will likely experience its anticoagulant effects to some extent. Aspirin irreversibly inhibits thromboxane production in platelets; thus, its anticoagulant effects will persist for 4 to 6 days (platelet life span) after ingestion. These effects are clinically significant in individuals with preexisting clotting disorders (hypoprothrombinemia, hemophilia, or thrombocytopenia) or in those taking prescription anticoagulants such as warfarin

(Coumadin)—therefore, salicylates should not be used in these instances.[16] For the same reason, salicylates are also contraindicated for individuals diagnosed with anemia. In addition, people who will undergo elective surgery, including some dental procedures, should refrain from using aspirin for at least 2 weeks before the surgical procedure to avoid excessive bleeding.

• Kidney damage, also known as *nephrotoxicity,* resulting from aspirin ingestion occurs mainly in elderly users, patients with congestive heart failure or preexisting kidney disorders, or people with a history of long-term aspirin use. Nephrotoxicity is rare among healthy athletes who only use aspirin for a few days. You should know, however, that aspirin can inhibit the excretion of uric acid; therefore, aspirin should not be used by anyone who has been diagnosed as having gout or who is already ingesting a prescription medication for the treatment of gout.[16]

• Hypersensitive individuals may experience an allergic reaction to aspirin, which generally takes the form of hives, edema, difficulty breathing, bronchospasm, rhinitis, or shock. Aspirin intolerance is serious but relatively rare, occurring most commonly only in patients with chronic hives (up to 28%), asthma (up to 19%), and nasal polyps (up to 23%). People with a history of aspirin intolerance may use acetaminophen, but they should avoid nonsteroidal anti-inflammatory drugs (NSAIDs)— such as ibuprofen and naproxen—which may cause a similar allergic reaction.[4]

• In children, aspirin has been linked to Reye's syndrome, an acute and potentially fatal illness that sometimes follows viral infections such as influenza and chicken pox. An exact mechanism has never been discovered to explain how aspirin use results in Reye's syndrome. However, since the use of aspirin as an antipyretic in children has greatly diminished over the past 20 years, Reye's syndrome has almost disappeared. Thus, for the relief of fever and other symptoms of viral infection, caregivers should give acetaminophen or ibuprofen rather than aspirin to anyone under the age of 18 years.[16]

Aspirin and other salicylates should be administered only as directed on the package label. An extreme overdose can cause depression of the central nervous system, resulting in respiratory failure, circulatory collapse, coma, and even death. Early warning signs of aspirin overdose include ringing in the ears, hearing loss, headache, rapid heartbeat, dizziness, and nausea. If such symptoms do not subside after discontinuing use, consult a physician. If black or bloody stools, abdominal pain, and vomiting of blood occur after ingesting aspirin, this may indicate gastrointestinal bleeding, so seek immediate medical attention.

Care should be taken to ensure that athletes are not ingesting too much aspirin. Aspirin and other salicylates are found in a variety of OTC products. Many cough and cold medications contain aspirin as a primary ingredient for pain relief, as do some medications for the relief of upset stomachs. Therefore, combining aspirin with these drugs may predispose patients to an excess amount of salicylate and possible toxicity. Bismuth subsalicylate (Pepto-Bismol) releases salicylate and could cause toxicity if used in combination with plain aspirin. Some salicylate derivatives are marketed as prescription-only drugs for the treatment of inflammatory bowel disease; these drugs should not be taken in combination with aspirin.

Use of aspirin and other salicylates should also be avoided in combination with any of the following substances:[16]

• Warfarin or other anticoagulants (increased risk of hemorrhage)

• Corticosteroids, such as dexamethasone, hydrocortisone, and prednisone (salicylates may reduce their effectiveness and increase the risk of gastrointestinal injury)

• Other salicylates or NSAIDs, including ibuprofen and naproxen (add-on effects may increase the risk of GI bleeding)

• Alcohol (i.e., ethanol; alcohol and aspirin can both cause direct injury to the gastric mucosa, resulting in an increased risk for GI bleeding)

Contraindications

In addition to the conditions already mentioned, aspirin and other salicylates are contraindicated for the following individuals:

• Pregnant women. Research has revealed that aspirin causes birth defects in animals and appears to increase the incidence of prolonged pregnancy, difficult delivery, stillbirths, and neonatal deaths. Thus, pregnant women should avoid ingesting aspirin, particularly during the last trimester.[16]

• People who have a history of peptic ulcer disease, GI bleeding, or liver disease.

- People who have nasal polyps.
- People who have a history of tartrazine dye sensitivity.
- People with asthma. One study found that aspirin-containing substances were likely to cause bronchospasm in susceptible individuals from minutes to hours after ingestion.[10]

Combination Aspirin Products

Since the initial synthesis of aspirin, researchers have sought to maintain its excellent efficacy but limit its side effects. The results include buffered aspirin, delayed-release aspirin, and aspirin with caffeine. These are described here to help you advise your athletes on what formulation may be the most helpful, depending on their specific needs.

- **Buffered aspirin.** Under certain circumstances, aspirin can invade the gastric mucosa, causing injury to the stomach lining. Thus, manufacturers may add buffering agents—principally antacid compounds that are alkaline—to aspirin in an attempt to neutralize stomach acid, thereby diminishing the chances of GI distress. When stomach contents are neutralized briefly, aspirin can dissolve and be absorbed into the bloodstream more rapidly, which speeds and prolongs pain relief. Although this theory sounds plausible, there is little scientific proof to support it. Buffered aspirin products may reduce the stomach distress that some people experience with plain aspirin, but they do not necessarily reduce the risk of gastrointestinal bleeding in susceptible individuals. Also, research has not shown that buffered aspirin provides faster or longer pain relief.[16]
- **Delayed-release aspirin.** Aspirin tablets labeled "timed release" or "delayed release" have a special coating that keeps the aspirin from dissolving in the stomach, thereby preventing the gastric irritation it can sometimes cause. The purpose of the coating is to delay dissolution of the tablets until they pass through the stomach and can be absorbed in the small intestine. But because it may sometimes take several hours for the tablets to reach the intestine, not only is dissolution delayed, so too is pain relief. Still, people who have experienced previous stomach upset after ingesting plain aspirin may find the delayed-release products somewhat more acceptable.[16]
- **Aspirin with caffeine.** Small amounts of the stimulant caffeine appear to enhance aspirin's analgesic effects, particularly in regard to headaches. The caffeine in these products both acts as a mood elevator and tightens the distended blood vessels that cause headache pain.[16] Anacin is an example of an OTC product containing both aspirin and caffeine.

NSAIDs

In the latter half of the 20th century, aspirin served as the prototype for the development of NSAIDs. The goal of this early research was to develop a medication that maintained aspirin's potent anti-inflammatory properties, but with limited side effects. Like aspirin, all NSAIDs inhibit the COX enzyme. However, unlike aspirin, the NSAIDs do not bind to the COX enzyme irreversibly—thus, certain effects, such as the antiplatelet action, are not as pronounced.

A major breakthrough was thought to have been achieved in the mid-1990s with the discovery of two COX isoenzymes. COX-1 was initially believed to be a "housekeeping" enzyme primarily present in platelets and the GI tract. In this role, COX-1 would be responsible for regulation of vascular hemostasis and gastric cytoprotection. COX-2 was thought to be primarily induced at sites of inflammation.[5]

With this discovery, pharmaceutical companies sought to develop medications that would selectively block only the COX-2 isoenzyme and have no effect on COX-1. Thus, they hoped to create the perfect aspirin derivative—a drug that inhibited inflammation but had no side effects such as prolonged bleeding or gastrointestinal irritation. With this promising potential, rofecoxib (Vioxx), celecoxib (Celebrex), and valdecoxib (Bextra) were aggressively marketed and quickly became some of the most widely prescribed medications during the early 2000s. Soon after their release, troubling data arose regarding increased risk for myocardial infarction in patients taking these medications. Rofecoxib and valdecoxib were withdrawn from the market in 2004.

A full overview of the risks for myocardial infarction with the long-term use of NSAIDs is beyond the scope of this text. The most current data suggest that there may be some cardiac risk for *all patients* taking *any* of the available NSAIDs, not just COX-2 selective inhibitors.[6] The risks are greater in older individuals with underlying cardiovascular disease. However, these recent findings show that NSAIDs are medications with many potential side effects. They also show us that the functions of the COX isoenzymes are much more complicated than originally believed. A physician must carefully weigh these potential side effects when deciding whether to prescribe a particular NSAID or to direct a patient to use an OTC medication.

The actions of nonsalicylate NSAIDs are similar to those of salicylates, although the inhibitory effects on platelet activation (a necessary step in coagulation) are shorter lived in people using NSAIDs than in those using aspirin.

In general, you should consider NSAIDs to be a single group of drugs.[1] However, you can differentiate according to (1) their availability without a prescription (OTC versus prescription) and (2) their duration of action. Table 3.1 summarizes these differences. Over-the-counter formulations of these drugs tend to have shorter-acting effects than formulations that are available by prescription only. At present, only three nonsalicylate NSAIDs are available without prescription: ibuprofen, ketoprofen, and naproxen sodium. Larger doses of these three drugs continue to be available only by prescription.

Researchers have found the anti-inflammatory properties of NSAIDs to be particularly effective for relief of pain associated with menstrual cramps and arthritis. At prescription doses, these drugs are safe, effective, and well regarded for the treatment of arthritis and other inflammatory disorders.

Indications and Uses

Like aspirin, NSAIDs possess anti-inflammatory, analgesic, antipyretic, and antiplatelet properties. For NSAIDs, however, the antiplatelet actions are much shorter lived than those of aspirin. The actual duration of analgesic and anti-inflammatory effects of NSAIDs depends on the specific drug.

Despite decades of widespread use, little scientific data exist to support or refute the use of NSAIDs for

Table 3.1   Availability and Duration of Action for Various NSAIDs

Generic name (trade name)	Duration of action	Rx or OTC
Celecoxib (Celebrex)	Long	Rx
Diclofenac (Cataflam, Voltaren)	Short	Rx
Etodolac (Lodine)	Short	Rx
Fenoprofen (Nalfon)	Short	Rx
Flurbiprofen (Ansaid)	Short	Rx
Ibuprofen (Advil, Motrin, Nuprin)	Short	Rx and OTC
Indomethacin (Indocin)	Intermediate	Rx
Ketoprofen (Orudis, Actron)	Short	Rx and OTC
Ketorolac (Toradol)	Short	Rx
Meclofenamate sodium (Meclomen)	Short	Rx
Mefenamic acid (Ponstel)	Short	Rx
Meloxicam (Mobic)	Long	Rx
Nabumetone (Relafen)	Long	Rx
Naproxen (Naprosyn, Naprelan)	Intermediate	Rx
Naproxen sodium (Anaprox, Aleve)	Intermediate	Rx and OTC
Oxaprozin (Daypro)	Long	Rx
Piroxicam (Feldene)	Very long	Rx
Sulindac (Clinoril)	Intermediate	Rx
Tolmetin (Tolectin)	Short	Rx

acute or chronic musculoskeletal conditions. The goal in using NSAIDs is to inhibit the inflammatory response, thereby decreasing inflammation, pain, and tissue damage. However, the inflammatory response is the first stage in healing of any injured tissue. Thus, theoretically, NSAID use could diminish the inflammatory response after injury and actually *delay* the healing process.

The potential for increased bleeding in the injured tissue must also be considered. The antiplatelet effects of NSAIDs, though not as pronounced as those of aspirin, may still contribute to increased bleeding following acute musculoskeletal injury. Although this is a theoretical concern, it has not been found to be a significant drawback to NSAID use based on anecdotal data. Unfortunately, there is no clear consensus based on high-level evidence regarding the use of NSAIDs for acute musculoskeletal conditions.

Given the lack of conclusive data on the proper timing of initiation or duration of NSAID use in athletes, these drugs should be used judiciously and with caution. Since medical professionals may differ in their experiences and beliefs regarding NSAIDs, you should talk to your team physician about his or her preferences regarding the use of both prescription and OTC NSAIDs. As always, potential interactions with other medications must be considered for all athletes. For older athletes, the small (but significant) cardiovascular risks of NSAID use must also be kept in mind.

In clinical medicine, practitioners use nonsalicylate NSAIDs to treat rheumatic and inflammatory conditions such as ankylosing spondylitis, bursitis, rheumatoid arthritis, and juvenile rheumatoid arthritis. These drugs are also used for relief of menstrual pain (dysmenorrhea), fever, headache (including migraine), and other nonspecific mild to moderate pain.

NSAIDs are not currently banned by any athletic governing bodies, but regulations are often subject to change. For a complete list of banned substances, contact the appropriate governing body.[12,14]

Routes of Administration

NSAIDs are almost always administered orally, most often in tablet, capsule, or caplet form. You may also purchase ibuprofen in liquid form for children or adults who have difficulty swallowing pills. Several NSAIDs are also available by prescription for ophthalmic administration to treat postoperative inflammation and the itching associated with allergic conjunctivitis.

Though not commercially marketed in the United States, topical formulations of some NSAIDs can be compounded by specially trained pharmacists in this country. Ketoprofen cream has been commercially available for several years in Europe and has been found to be a safe and effective analgesic when applied to painful joints and muscle.[9]

General Dose Protocols

Ibuprofen was the first NSAID—and one of the first new pain relievers in 50 years—that the FDA made available over the counter. OTC ibuprofen products are generally formulated in 200 mg tablets or capsules. For adults, the recommended dose is two tablets (400 mg) every 4 to 6 hours, with a 24-hour maximum dose not to exceed 1,200 mg.[16] Liquid and chewable tablet formulations of ibuprofen are now available for administration to children. The specific dosage can be determined by comparing the child's age and weight and consulting the product label.

Naproxen sodium (Aleve) is longer acting than ibuprofen and is widely available in 220 mg capsules and tablets. The recommended dose is one tablet every 8 to 12 hours, with the 24-hour maximum dose not to exceed three tablets (660 mg).

Ketoprofen (Orudis KT and Actron) is the most potent of the NSAIDs currently available over the counter. Typically, manufacturers formulate the drug in 12.5 mg tablets; the recommended effective dose is one tablet every 4 to 6 hours. People who do not experience some relief from pain or fever within 1 hour of ingesting the first tablet may take a second tablet; however, no one should take more than two tablets every 4 to 6 hours. The FDA has set the maximum 24-hour dose of OTC ketoprofen at 75 mg (six tablets).

Unless otherwise directed by a physician, adults should limit their use of NSAIDs to 3 days for relief of fever and 10 days for relief of pain. Pain or fever that does not respond to an NSAID within these recommended time frames may be a sign of a more serious condition requiring medical attention.

Side Effects and Adverse Reactions

NSAIDs have potential side effects similar to those of aspirin, with a few exceptions.[1,13] For example, the antiplatelet effects of nonsalicylate NSAIDs are shorter lived than those of aspirin. NSAIDs may be a little easier on the stomach, too; in general, gastrointestinal bleeding seems to occur less frequently in nonsalicylate NSAID users than in aspirin users.[16]

As discussed, both the traditional NSAIDs and the newer COX-2 selective NSAIDs have been found to increase the risk of myocardial infarction in certain patients.[6] More studies are sure to provide additional information on this issue in the coming years, so you must stay updated on this important topic.

Nephrotoxicity has been associated with NSAID use, but primarily only in people with preexisting kidney disorders. In addition, NSAIDs may decrease the effectiveness of some antihypertensives.

Patients who are intolerant of aspirin are often also intolerant of nonsalicylate NSAIDs. Hypersensitive individuals may experience an anaphylactic reaction—hives, rash, intensive itching, and bronchospasm. If any of these symptoms occur in connection with NSAID ingestion, seek immediate medical attention. People with known sensitivity to aspirin should avoid NSAIDs as well; for them, acetaminophen is a safer choice for pain relief.

Researchers consider NSAIDs to be relatively safe when used as directed. However, because some combination products for relief of pain, fever, cough, and cold symptoms contain NSAIDs, users must take care to avoid an overdose. Symptoms of NSAID overdose are similar to those of aspirin overdose: diminished hearing, ringing in the ears, headache, dizziness, and nausea.[16] If symptoms such as these do not subside by discontinuing the drug, consult a doctor.

The following conditions may be signs of NSAID toxicity: difficulty breathing, rapid or irregular heartbeat, black or tarry stools, blood in the urine, photosensitivity, and jaundice (yellowing of the eyes or skin). If any such symptoms occur, seek immediate medical attention.

Contraindications

Encourage your athletes to use NSAIDs cautiously or to avoid them altogether in all the same situations as described for aspirin and other salicylates. In general, NSAIDs should not be used in combination with corticosteroids, anticoagulant drugs, aspirin, or other salicylates. Make sure your athletes are aware that they must be careful not to combine NSAID use with alcohol consumption. Drinking alcohol while taking NSAIDs greatly increases the risk of gastritis and GI bleeding.[3,11] Finally, pregnant women should avoid NSAIDs unless otherwise directed by a physician.

A handful of studies have raised concern over the effects of NSAID use on the healing of fractures. Based on the current available evidence, no firm recommendations can be made endorsing or prohibiting the use of NSAIDs in routine fracture management. Theoretically, NSAIDs may delay the healing of fractures. This effect could be magnified in an environment where healing is already compromised, such as with chronic illness, smoking, or a stress fracture of a bone with a poor blood supply (e.g., proximal fifth metatarsal, tarsal navicular). A review of the current literature indicates that the use of oral NSAIDs at appropriate doses is not contraindicated for early care of acute fractures in athletes.[7]

Appropriate and effective pain control in the acute phase of the inflammatory process must be considered. Many patients may be willing to accept the theoretical risk of a delay in their return to full function if they have adequate analgesia during the acute phase of the injury. This same scenario may be unacceptable for an athlete.

Guidelines for the Athletic Trainer

NSAIDs and aspirin are appropriate for many uses. But before recommending either to an athlete, you should consider the following:

• The acuity of the injury should be taken into account. As previously discussed, for acute injuries, an NSAID or aspirin may not be the best choice. You should discourage long-term use of anti-inflammatory medications in order to reduce the risk of an adverse reaction. Also, the condition in question may require medical attention if it does not resolve itself during 3 to 10 days of self-medication (10 days for pain; 3 days for fever).

• Certain conditions might preclude the use of NSAIDs or aspirin. You must always balance the benefit of taking an anti-inflammatory medication before strenuous exercise against the increased risk of gastrointestinal injury.

• Athletic trainers and team physicians have long been aware of athletes' using NSAIDs as a preventive measure before practices and games to control pain. This was confirmed by a recent study of 681 high school football players, which found that 15% used NSAIDs daily.[14] You should warn athletes against this practice because they may be exceeding recommended dosages and putting themselves at risk for serious side effects.

- Aspirin use is specifically contraindicated in athletes under the age of 18 years who have fever and in any athlete taking an anticoagulant, such as warfarin.

References and Resources

1. Brooks, P.M., and R.O. Day. 1991. Nonsteroidal anti-inflammatory drugs: Differences and similarities. *The New England Journal of Medicine* 324(24):1716-1725.

2. Burger, A. 1986. *Drugs and people: Medications, their history and origins, and the way they act.* Charlottesville, Virginia: University Press of Virginia.

3. Cooper, B.T., S.A. Douglas, L.A. Firth, J.A. Hannagan, and V.S. Chadwick. 1987. Erosive gastritis and gastrointestinal bleeding in a female runner. *Gastroenterology* 92(6):2019-2023.

4. Covington, T.R., R.R. Berardi, and L.L. Young, eds. 1993. *Handbook of nonprescription drugs.* 10th ed. Washington, D.C.: American Pharmaceutical Association.

5. Davies, N.M., and N.M. Skjodt. 2000. Choosing the right nonsteroidal anti-inflammatory drug for the right patient. *Clinical Pharmacokinetics* 38:377.

6. Graham, D.J. 2006. COX-2 inhibitors, other NSAIDs, and cardiovascular risk: The seduction of common sense. *JAMA* 296(13):1653-1656.

7. Koester, M.C., and K.P. Spindler. 2005. NSAIDs and fracture healing: What's the evidence? *Curr Sports Med Rep* 4(6) (December):289-290.

8. Mangus, B.C., and M.G. Miller. 2005. *Pharmacology application in athletic training.* Philadelphia: FA Davis.

9. Mason, L., R.A. Moore, J.E. Edwards, S. Derry, and H.J. McQuay. 2004. Topical NSAIDs for acute pain: A meta-analysis. *BMC Fam Pract* (May):10.

10. McDonald, J.R., D.A. Mathison, and D.D. Stevenson. 1972. Aspirin intolerance in asthma. *Journal of Allergy and Clinical Immunology* 50(4):198-207.

11. McMahon, L.F. Jr., M.J. Ryan, D. Larson, and R.L. Fisher. 1984. Occult gastrointestinal blood loss in marathon runners. *Annals of Internal Medicine* 100(6) (June):846-847.

12. National Collegiate Athletic Association. NCAA banned drug classes. www1.ncaa.org/membership/ed_outreach/health-safety/drug_testing/banned_drug_classes.pdf. Accessed 10/14/06.

13. NSAID overview. 1996. *Clinical pharmacology: An electronic drug reference and teaching guide.* Version 1.6. Gainesville, FL: Gold Standard Multimedia, Inc.

14. World Anti-Doping Agency. The world anti-doping code: The 2006 prohibited list. www.wada-ama.org/rtecontent/document/2006_LIST.pdf. Accessed 10/14/06.

15. Warner, D.C., G. Schnepf, M.S. Barrett, D. Dian, and N.L. Swigonski. 2002. Prevalence, attitudes, and behaviors related to the use of nonsteroidal anti-inflammatory drugs (NSAIDs) in student athletes. *J Adolesc Health* 30:150.

16. Zimmerman, D.R. 1992. *Zimmerman's complete guide to nonprescription drugs.* 2nd ed. Detroit: Gale Research.

CHAPTER 4

Anti-Inflammatory Drugs: Corticosteroids

Steroid hormones are lipid soluble. They have a chemical structure similar to cholesterol, and many are derived directly from cholesterol. Corticosteroids are steroid hormones produced within the adrenal cortex (or synthetic versions of these hormones manufactured within a laboratory). Four types of corticosteroids are produced by the adrenal cortex: mineralocorticoids (aldosterone), glucocorticoids (cortisol), androgens, and estrogens.

Corticosteroids should not be confused with anabolic steroids, which are derivatives of the male reproductive hormone testosterone. As you probably know, exogenous (artificially produced) testosterone is sometimes used by athletes as a performance-enhancing drug to increase muscle size and strength. Although both substances are called *steroids*, the actions and origins of corticosteroids and anabolic steroids are quite different.[4]

Indications and Uses

In clinical medicine, practitioners use corticosteroids to treat dozens of conditions, ranging from a simple skin rash to asthma. Corticosteroids are powerful drugs, and when administered systemically, they may affect almost all of the body's organ systems. Therefore, these drugs must be used only when indicated.

The majority of corticosteroids are available only by prescription. Only topical hydrocortisone is available over the counter. Topical hydrocortisone is used to treat external itching and inflammation associated with fungal infections such as athlete's foot, jock itch, ringworm, and candidiasis. You

KEY TERMS

anabolic steroids

bursitis

corticosteroids

glucocorticoid

hydrocortisone

steroid

should note that hydrocortisone is not an antifungal; it is merely effective in relieving the irritation. In fact, prescription-strength topical steroids may actually worsen fungal infections if used instead of an antifungal. (For more information about topical antifungals, see chapter 8.)

Corticosteroids are typically prescribed for the following conditions:

- Skin disorders, including psoriasis, eczema, and other diseases

- Nasal inflammation, including allergic rhinitis and nonallergic disorders of the nasal passages

- Respiratory ailments, such as asthma

- Inflammatory musculoskeletal disorders, including rheumatoid arthritis and bursitis

- Gastrointestinal disorders, such as ulcerative colitis and Crohn's disease

In sports medicine, practitioners primarily use corticosteroids for the treatment of bursitis and inflamed joints that are unresponsive to NSAIDs, as well as for conditions such as asthma, exercise-induced bronchospasm, and allergic rhinitis.[2] Topical corticosteroids are used to relieve external itching and minor skin irritations.

Corticosteroids are among the most complex drugs used to treat humans. Corticosteroids exert their influence by reacting with receptors in the cytoplasm of affected cells; in turn, the resulting steroid-receptor complex affects RNA transcription of selected genes. Researchers believe that the anti-inflammatory action of corticosteroids is a result of the drug interfering—through a complex process—with the ability of leukocytes to migrate into affected areas. Specifically, corticosteroids appear to suppress the release of chemotactic (chemical movement) factors that mediate the body's inflammatory response.

Corticosteroid injection therapy for the treatment of inflamed joints first gained popularity in the early 1950s. The theory behind using steroids for this purpose appears to be based on their anti-inflammatory properties. Injured tissues incite an inflammatory response in the body, resulting in local tissue edema and subsequent swelling, pain, and limited motion. An anti-inflammatory agent such as a corticosteroid will potentially block this response.[7]

Research shows that corticosteroids—in addition to blocking the body's natural response to inflammation—also inhibit collagen synthesis. The fact that these two inhibitory properties of corticosteroids cannot be separated from one another presents a problem with regard to tissue healing. Since inflammation—the first phase of soft tissue healing—is inhibited by corticosteroids, the overall healing process is delayed. However, collagen synthesis appears to recover over time, so this delay appears reversible.[7]

The many ways that the body handles corticosteroids are too complex to summarize in this text. You should know, however, that corticosteroids are lipid-soluble compounds, readily stored by the body. Thus, their effects can last for days or weeks.

Routes of Administration

Corticosteroids are available as topical creams and ointments; nasal inhalants and sprays; lung (oral) inhalants and sprays; tablets and syrups for oral ingestion; and solutions for intra-articular, bursal, or tendon sheath injection. The most appropriate form of administration depends on the condition that the drug is intended to treat. All corticosteroids, with the exception of topical hydrocortisone, require a prescription.

Corticosteroids administered by oral inhalation for the treatment of asthma and other respiratory ailments include the following:

- Beclomethasone oral inhalation (QVAR)
- Budesonide inhalation solution (Pulmicort Respules)
- Budesonide oral inhalation (Pulmicort Turbuhaler)
- Flunisolide oral inhalation (Aerobid-M, Aerobid)
- Fluticasone inhalation aerosol (Flovent)
- Fluticasone powder for oral inhalation (Flovent Rotadisk)
- Mometasone inhalation powder (Asmanex Twisthaler)
- Triamcinolone oral inhalation (Azmacort)

Corticosteroids administered by nasal inhalation for the treatment of nasal inflammation and allergic rhinitis include the following:

- Beclomethosone (Benconase, Beconase AQ, Vancenase, Vancenase AQ, Vancenase Pockethaler)
- Budesonide (Rhinocort)
- Flunisolide (Nasarel)
- Fluticasone (Flonase)
- Triamcinolone (Nasacort, Nasacort AQ, Tri-Nasal)
- Mometasone (Nasonex)

Corticosteroids administered by injection for the treatment of arthritis, bursitis, and other inflammatory conditions include the following:

- Betamethasone (Celestone)
- Dexamethasone (Decadron)
- Hydrocortisone (Solu-Cortef)
- Methylprednisolone (Depo-Medrol)
- Prednisolone (Hydeltrasol)
- Triamcinolone (Aristospan, Kenalog-10, Kenalog-40)

Prescribers may also use prednisone, an orally administered corticosteroid, to treat inflammatory conditions such as rheumatoid arthritis, ulcerative colitis, and Crohn's disease. Topically administered corticosteroids include hydrocortisone and hydrocortisone acetate.

Side Effects and Adverse Reactions

Corticosteroids are extremely potent drugs, especially when administered systemically. Their beneficial effects are dramatic, but chronic use of corticosteroids can produce significant side effects. Reports of adverse reactions to corticosteroids are numerous, and many are quite serious. As an athletic trainer, you must be able to identify the more common side effects, and you must know whether these complications appear immediately or only after long-term administration.

Although corticosteroids in the form of topical creams and nasal or oral inhalants rarely produce systemic effects over the short term, the body may systemically absorb such products during prolonged use. Corticosteroids administered by intra-articular injection may also produce adverse systemic and local effects. Systemic effects include a transient (12- to 24-hour) rise in blood sugar in patients with diabetes, as well as facial flushing (warm feeling accompanied by redness of the skin). Locally, pain 1 to 2 hours following the injection, skin hypopigmentation, and local tissue atrophy may also occur. In addition, there is always a risk of infection (though rare) following any type of joint injection.

Corticosteroid injections into and around tendons are occasionally used. Most commonly, these injections are used to treat lateral epicondylitis.[4] Injections into and around the patellar and Achilles tendons are contraindicated because of concerns about increased risk for tendon rupture following injection. It is hypothesized that the corticosteroid's inhibition of healing in the tendon tissue may contribute to tendon rupture.[4]

Unfortunately, prolonged oral use of corticosteroids may suppress the body's immune system, making the user more susceptible to opportunistic infections. Moreover, these drugs can mask the symptoms of an infection. By the time the user actually notices symptoms, the infection may have entered an advanced stage that is more difficult to treat.

Prolonged use can also increase an individual's risk of developing osteoporosis, cataracts, glaucoma, Cushing's syndrome ("moon face"), and diabetes. Osteonecrosis of the femoral and humeral heads has also been reported following corticosteroid use. Any individual who has had a course of oral corticosteroids and complains of shoulder or hip pain should be reevaluated by his or her physician. However, people who are using corticosteroids for more than 2 weeks should not stop the drugs suddenly. Use of corticosteroids will often cause production in the adrenal glands to greatly diminish, and the body will be unable to immediately restart production. Thus, an abrupt cessation of corticosteroid use may result in adrenal insufficiency. Experts recommend a withdrawal period during which dosages are gradually reduced to avoid serious adverse reactions.[6]

Systemic corticosteroids carry an increased risk of provoking gastrointestinal (GI) ulceration when combined with alcohol or NSAIDs (including aspirin). In general, patients receiving corticosteroids by inhalation or intra-articular injection do not need to be concerned about gastrointestinal complications.

Reactions to topical corticosteroids closely resemble the conditions these products are designed to treat. These side effects include mild and transient skin rash, burning, irritation, dryness, redness, itching, and scaling. Such symptoms are not serious and usually abate soon after discontinuing use of the product.[9]

Other forms of corticosteroids may cause stomach upset, changes in appetite (either increase or decrease), restlessness, dizziness, sleeplessness, change in skin color, and unusual hair growth on the face or body. Physicians do not consider these reactions serious, but you or the athlete should nevertheless bring them to the attention of a physician to prevent further complications if the individual continues to use the drug.[6]

The more serious side effects of corticosteroid use include the following:[6]

- Optic effects—eye pain, loss of or blurred vision

- Gastrointestinal effects—stomach pain or burning; black, tarry stools (secondary to gastrointestinal bleeding); nausea and vomiting

- Circulatory effects—swelling of feet and legs; generalized fluid retention (edema); unusual bruising

- Skin reactions—severe and lasting skin rash, hives, or burning, itching, painful skin; blisters, acne, or other skin eruptions

- Menstrual irregularities

- Prolonged sore throat, fever, cold, or other signs of infection

Some side effects may be associated with specific types of corticosteroids. However, many of the common reactions occur in connection with all corticosteroids, but you will not see all of the reactions for all routes of administration. Table 4.1 lists the most common side effects for the various routes of administration.

The most serious side effects of corticosteroid use are associated with orally ingested substances that produce a systemic reaction. Most athletes do not suffer from chronic inflammatory diseases that require oral corticosteroids; therefore, as an athletic trainer, you will seldom encounter a systemic corticosteroid reaction. As previously discussed, short-term use of a corticosteroid by inhalation (oral or nasal), which is more common among athletes, rarely produces a systemic effect.

Considerations Before Use

By reducing inflammation, corticosteroids may theoretically delay or retard pain that limits exercise. Unfortunately, chronic use of these drugs is associated with several major adverse reactions, including osteonecrosis (destruction or death of bone tissue) and immunosuppression.[1]

You should ensure that your athletes avoid corticosteroids in combination with any of the following health conditions: HIV or AIDS; heart disease; hypertension; diabetes; diverticulitis, gastritis, or peptic ulcer disease; glaucoma or cataracts; liver or kidney disease; tuberculosis; lupus; or any infections, such as a cold or flu.[6]

Studies have found that inhaled corticosteroids generally have no significant effect on the levels of naturally occurring testosterone in blood and therefore do not affect the testosterone test results used in judging anabolic steroid abuse.[1] However, researchers have found that long-term use of orally ingested corticosteroids (e.g., prednisone) reduces the plasma concentration of testosterone by as much as 33%.[1] The NCAA and WADA have different regulations regarding the use of corticosteroids, and these regulations are subject to change. For a complete list of banned substances, contact the appropriate governing body.[5,8]

Guidelines for the Athletic Trainer

- Athletes who have been prescribed a corticosteroid inhaler (such as beclomethasone or triamcinolone) to treat asthma should use the drug only as prescribed. It should not be used in the case of an acute asthma exacerbation.

- An athlete who has recently received an intra-articular injection of a corticosteroid should not stress the involved joint too soon. The injection may mask any pain that might otherwise serve as a warning to limit movement or weight-bearing activities. Naturally, placing stress on the injured joint before it has had a chance to heal could result in further injury.

- In general, corticosteroids inhibit collagen synthesis, delaying the healing of wounds. This is not a concern with intra-articular injections.

Table 4.1   Common Side Effects of Corticosteroids

Route of administration	Potential side effects	Onset
Oral inhalation	Coughing	Immediate
	Dysphonia (hoarseness)	Immediate
	Oral candidiasis (yeast infection)	Delayed
Nasal inhalation	Local irritation	Immediate
Intra-articular injection	Pain in the joint	Immediate
	Infection	Immediate
Bursa injection	Infection	Immediate
Tendon injection	Tendon rupture	Delayed

However, injections in and around certain tendons should be avoided because of concerns about possible tendon rupture.

• With the exception of topical hydrocortisone, corticosteroids are available only by prescription. Athletes receiving these substances by any other route of administration—whether by oral or nasal inhalation, ingestion, or injection—should be under the care of a medical doctor.

References and Resources

1. Fuentes, R.J., J.M. Rosenberg, and A. Davis. 1996. *Athletic drug reference '96*. Research Triangle Park, NC: Clean Data.

2. Kobayashi, R.H., and M.B. Million. 1991. Exercise-induced asthma, anaphylaxis, and urticaria. *Primary Care* 18(4):809-831.

3. Leadbetter, W.B. 1995. Anti-inflammatory therapy in sports injury: The role of nonsteroidal drugs and corticosteroid injection. *Clin Sports Med* 14(2):353-410.

4. Mutschler, E., and H. Derendorf. 1994. *Basic and applied principles of drug actions*. Boca Raton, FL: CRC Press.

5. National Collegiate Athletic Association. NCAA banned drug classes. www1.ncaa.org/membership/ed_outreach/health-safety/drug_testing/banned_drug_classes.pdf. Accessed 10/14/06.

6. Time-Life Books, eds. 1996. *The medical advisor: The complete guide to alternative and conventional treatments*. Alexandria, VA: Time-Life.

7. Wiggins, M.E., P.D. Fadale, H. Barrach, M.G. Ehrlich, and W.R. Walsh. 1994. Healing characteristics of a type I collagenous structure treated with corticosteroids. *The American Journal of Sports Medicine* 22(2):279.

8. World Anti-Doping Agency. The world anti-doping code: The 2006 prohibited list. www.wada-ama.org/rtecontent/document/2006_LIST.pdf. Accessed 10/14/06.

9. Zimmerman, D.R. 1992. *Zimmerman's complete guide to nonprescription drugs*. 2nd ed. Detroit: Gale Research.

CHAPTER 5

Non-Anti-Inflammatory Systemic Analgesics

Like the salicylates and NSAIDs discussed in previous chapters, analgesic drugs classified as non-anti-inflammatory agents relieve pain and fever, but there is one important distinction: Non-anti-inflammatory analgesics act to alleviate pain independently of any anti-inflammatory effect. Consequently, although these drugs do exert analgesic effects, they may be less useful in the treatment of inflammatory conditions such as rheumatoid arthritis, bursitis, and tenosynovitis.[1]

Non-anti-inflammatory drugs are available in both prescription and nonprescription strengths. The most widely used drug among these analgesics—acetaminophen (Tylenol)—may be purchased over the counter. Most other common non-anti-inflammatory analgesics are narcotics, which individuals can only obtain by prescription. Although the term *narcotic* actually refers to any drug that dulls the senses and induces sleep, narcotic analgesics are those that specifically alter a person's sense of pain. Typically, these drugs are opiate agonists, substances derived from opium that act by stimulating a specific receptor to produce a desired response—in this case, a decreased awareness of pain.

Non-anti-inflammatory analgesics can be further categorized by the degree of pain they best relieve:

- Acetaminophen (Tylenol): for mild to moderate pain
- Opiate agonists
  - Codeine: for mild to moderate pain unrelieved by nonopiates
  - Meperidine: for moderate to severe pain
  - Morphine: for severe pain

- Tramadol (Ultram): for mild to moderate pain
- Combination products (Fiorinal, Tylenol with codeine): for mild to moderate pain

Although all non-anti-inflammatory analgesics have the same purpose (pain relief), the different types accomplish that purpose by very different means. Opiate agonists dull pain awareness by stimulating specific opiate receptors throughout the body's central nervous system.[7] Tramadol curbs pain in two ways. It can act as a weak agonist for one type of opiate receptor. It can also inhibit the reuptake of the neurotransmitters norepinephrine and serotonin, thus reducing pain awareness.[8] Tramadol is a synthetic analog of codeine (i.e., it is similar in structure but different in respect to elemental composition); however, tramadol has a lower affinity (attraction) for opioid receptors than codeine does. Acetaminophen's analgesic mechanism of action is unknown.

Indications and Uses

Like aspirin and NSAIDs, acetaminophen is routinely used for the relief of mild to moderate pain and fever. Using acetaminophen has several advantages. For example, people who are allergic to aspirin will find acetaminophen to be a tolerable alternative for pain relief—so, too, will people who have experienced stomach distress associated with aspirin or other salicylates. Acetaminophen does not cause gastrointestinal bleeding, nor does it interfere with the drugs that are typically prescribed for the treatment of gout.

However, because acetaminophen is metabolized by the liver, people whose livers are damaged or diseased or who are heavy consumers of alcohol should not use this drug. Overdoses can cause hepatotoxicity and even death in people who have liver disease.

Opiate agonists—codeine, meperidine, and morphine—are narcotic drugs that act on the central nervous system to alter the perception of pain. Practitioners typically use them to treat moderate to severe pain that does not respond to other non-anti-inflammatory analgesics. Opiate agonists may sometimes be combined with nonnarcotic analgesics, such as aspirin and acetaminophen. In addition, physicians prescribe meperidine and morphine to relieve severe pain associated with some types of cancer and other debilitating conditions. Because of their potential to cause dependency in chronic users, opiate agonists are classified as controlled substances, and physicians generally use them with caution.

Tramadol, which is available only by prescription, is a relatively new addition to the arsenal of non-anti-inflammatory analgesics. Although widely used in Europe since the late 1970s, this drug did not receive FDA approval for use in the United States until early 1995. Tramadol is equivalent in potency to meperidine, an opiate derivative. Physicians use tramadol primarily to control moderate pain.[8]

Routes of Administration

Non-anti-inflammatory analgesics are typically administered orally in tablet or capsule form. Acetaminophen is also available as a liquid for children or adults who have difficulty swallowing pills. Rectal suppositories are available for the administration of acetaminophen to people who are vomiting, unconscious, or otherwise unable to ingest the drug orally. Tramadol and most opiate agonists are administered by mouth. In cases of severe pain, opiate agonists such as morphine and meperidine may be administered intravenously or by intramuscular injection for faster relief. Patients with chronic severe pain can benefit from a transdermal opiate administered through the use of a patch applied to the skin. This method of delivery allows for a more stable concentration of medication in the bloodstream—and for better pain control.

All the analgesics described in this chapter take effect within 30 to 60 minutes of oral administration, but effects are much faster when the drug is administered by IV or intramuscular injection. The effects of most non-anti-inflammatory analgesics last 3 to 4 hours, although some opiate agonists may last for a longer or shorter duration. Consult the label on OTC products (acetaminophen) or ask a pharmacist for specific information about dose size, frequency, and duration of action.

General Dose Protocols

Acetaminophen is typically formulated in 325 mg tablets, capsules, or caplets. For adults, the recommended dose is two tablets (650 mg) every 4 hours. Acetaminophen is also available over the counter in larger doses (usually labeled "extra strength" or "maximum strength"); individuals should only take these 500 mg tablets or capsules every 6 hours. In either case, the 24-hour maximum dose of acetaminophen should not exceed 4,000 mg.[10] Still, since manufacturers formulate their products in varying strengths, you should make sure that athletes check the label for specific dose instructions before ingesting any acetaminophen tablets.

Less potent formulations of acetaminophen are available for administration to children. Specific doses of children's acetaminophen products are determined by age and weight, so consult product labels for the correct dose.

Dosage protocols for opiate agonists depend on the potency and content of the specific substance. Read and follow all label directions and refer any questions about a specific drug to the pharmacist or prescribing physician.

Tramadol is typically administered in doses of 50 to 100 mg every 4 to 6 hours, with a 24-hour maximum dose not to exceed 400 mg. For initial pain relief, 50 mg doses may be sufficient, but 100 mg doses are generally more effective.[8]

Side Effects and Adverse Reactions

Analgesic medications are widely used and are considered quite safe. However, a variety of potential complications must be considered when an athlete is using a pain-relieving medication. Some common side effects that may result from the use of analgesic medications are listed in table 5.1.

Acetaminophen

When used as directed, acetaminophen is considered to be one of the safest over-the-counter medications on the market today. Unlike aspirin and NSAIDs, this pain reliever will not result in gastric irritation or bleeding. It can, however, have detrimental effects on the liver, especially in cases of severe overdose or even when normal doses are taken every day for several weeks. In addition, research has shown that subjects who take acetaminophen in combination with alcohol or while fasting are at a higher-than-average risk for developing hepatotoxicity.[6,11] In people who are too sick to eat, even moderate doses of acetaminophen can result in severe liver damage, leading to convulsions, coma, and death.[10] Acetaminophen has no apparent effects on athletic performance and therefore is safe to use before exercise.

Acetaminophen overdose is serious and can be life threatening; treatment must start within 24 hours to avoid permanent liver damage. Symptoms of overdose include nausea, vomiting, increased sweating, loss of appetite, and abdominal pain. If any such symptoms occur in combination with acetaminophen therapy, seek medical treatment immediately.

Opiate Agonists

When used as directed and for a limited period of time, opiate agonists (codeine, meperidine, morphine, and the like) are considered quite safe. Adverse reactions are similar for all types of opiate agonists. The only differences are in the intensity of the effect, which is primarily a function of the individual drug's dose and duration of action. The most worrisome adverse reaction to opiate agonists involves depression of functions in the central nervous system (CNS) or depression of respiratory functions. These conditions are unlikely to occur, however, unless the athlete ingests excessive doses of the drug or combines it with another CNS depressant such as alcohol.

Serious adverse reactions to opiate agonists are characterized by slow, shallow breathing; skin rash, hives, or itching; facial swelling; decrease in blood pressure or heart rate; rapid heartbeat accompanied by increased sweating and shortness of breath; severe constipation; and nausea, stomach pain, or vomiting. If any such symptoms occur in connection with the use of an opiate agonist, you should tell the athlete to stop taking the drug and seek medical attention. In general, opiate agonists should not be taken by people with a history of convulsions or drug abuse, inflammatory bowel disease, kidney or liver impairment, breathing problems, hypothyroidism, bladder or prostate problems, or gallbladder disease.[7]

Less serious side effects associated with using opiate agonists include dry mouth, drowsiness, mild nausea, mild constipation, difficulty in urinating, and frequent urge to urinate. If symptoms persist, the athlete should consult a physician.

Table 5.1   Common Side Effects and Adverse Reactions From Using Analgesics

Medication	Route	Potential side effects or adverse reactions
Acetaminophen	Oral or rectal	Liver toxicity
Opiate agonists	Oral	Respiratory depression Constipation Nausea Tolerance or dependency
Tramadol	Oral	Dependency Increased seizure risk*

*in patients taking antidepressant medications or who have a preexisting seizure disorder

Repeated or prolonged use of an opiate agonist may lead to the development of tolerance to the drug's therapeutic and nontherapeutic effects; as a result, the athlete may require larger and more frequent doses of the drug for relief of pain. Chronic use of opiate agonists followed by abrupt discontinuation leads to withdrawal syndrome. Symptoms of withdrawal syndrome include fever, runny nose or sneezing, diarrhea, goose flesh, unusually large pupils, nervousness or irritability, and rapid heartbeat.[7] Athletes who have been taking opiate agonists on a regular basis or who have been taking large doses for a few days should consult a physician before they stop taking the drug.

Opiate agonists should not be used before exercise or athletic activity because they may cause drowsiness, which in turn may impair hand–eye coordination. In addition, since all analgesics increase the pain threshold, an athlete under the influence of any painkiller—prescription or otherwise—may fail to recognize a serious injury when it occurs. Users may therefore perceive serious situations as safe, thereby placing themselves and their fellow competitors at risk of injury.[2]

Tramadol

Tramadol (Ultram) is a relatively new drug with a unique dual mechanism of action. As mentioned, it exerts agonistic properties at opiate receptors and interferes with neurotransmitter reuptake. The manufacturer originally promoted tramadol as having no potential for inducing physical dependence; however, the manufacturer has since withdrawn this claim.[5] The manufacturer now recommends that the drug not be used by patients with a history of opiate addiction or dependency.

Aside from dependency, the most significant problem with tramadol appears to be a small risk that it may induce seizures in patients taking antidepressant medications or patients who have a preexisting seizure disorder.[8] You should ensure that such people avoid this drug. Since tramadol has many pharmacological actions similar to those of opiate agonists, this substance should be used cautiously during competition (until research reveals its effects clearly and completely).

Combination Products

Because dozens of combination products—each with slightly different ingredients—are currently on the market, it would be impossible to summarize the potential adverse effects of these drugs. You should strive to determine the active ingredients of any combination analgesics (narcotic or otherwise) that your athletes are taking so that you can help them avoid or recognize adverse reactions.

Combination drugs containing salicylates are of special concern. If taken by themselves and only as directed for short periods of time, salicylates rarely cause nephrotoxicity.

Considerations Before Use

The following sections summarize the precautions you should teach your athletes to consider when using non-anti-inflammatory drugs. Be aware that you will probably have the most trouble convincing your athletes that acetaminophen can have side effects; this drug has a well-deserved reputation for being extremely safe—but only in recommended doses for short-term use.

The NCAA and WADA have different regulations regarding the use of analgesic medications, and these regulations are subject to change. For a complete list of banned substances, contact the appropriate governing body.[4,9]

Acetaminophen

Acetaminophen is a relatively safe analgesic. It does not cause drowsiness, nor does it appear to affect athletic performance. Acetaminophen is not banned by any governing body at this time. Because of its link to hepatotoxicity, however, acetaminophen should not be used by anyone whose liver is diseased or damaged or even by healthy individuals for prolonged periods of time. People who regularly consume alcohol should also avoid this substance.

Even in normal doses, acetaminophen can cause adverse reactions when used regularly over many weeks or months. Several over-the-counter combination products for the treatment of pain, fever, colds, and coughs contain acetaminophen. To help your athletes avoid a possible overdose, you should encourage them to read product labels carefully and to heed all warnings about drug interaction before ingesting any combination product.

Opiate Agonists

Opiate agonists act as depressants to the body's respiratory and CNS functions. Because the depressant effects of one agent will add on to those of another, you should insist that your athletes avoid combinations of these drugs. In addition, people taking opiate agonists should avoid other depressant substances, including muscle relaxants, antihistamines, and alcohol.

All opiate agonists cause drowsiness, and none should be used by athletes competing in events that involve throwing, catching, or shooting. The USOC bans all opiate agonists except codeine and dihydrocodeine; the NCAA only bans heroin (under the broad classification of "street drugs").[2]

Tramadol

Because it may cause seizures, tramadol should not be administered to anyone who is already taking an antidepressant or anticonvulsant medication. Also, people who have demonstrated prior hypersensitivity to an opiate agonist should not be given tramadol.[5]

Combination Products

Combination products are particularly tricky to monitor because each one contains different ingredients in varying amounts. To avoid adverse reactions or an overdose of any one ingredient, you and your athletes should be sure to check the contents of a combination product before ingesting it along with other medications. If an athlete is taking a combination product that contains acetaminophen, you should warn him or her about taking additional acetaminophen because the additional dose may cause acetaminophen toxicity. Some combination products contain caffeine, which researchers have shown to have ergogenic properties. So keep in mind that excessive quantities of caffeine are banned by the NCAA[4] and WADA[9] and may affect an athlete's eligibility status for competitive events.[2]

Muscle Relaxants

Muscle relaxants are widely prescribed by physicians for a variety of conditions, particularly low back injuries, even though the therapeutic efficacy of these drugs is questioned.[3] The exact mechanism of muscle relaxants is not known, but they do not act directly on the muscle fibers. Instead, they may cause a mild general sedative effect, producing overall relaxation of the body. The sedative effect may allow the injured individual to relax, rest, and sleep, secondarily reducing muscle spasm. Muscle relaxants are often used in conjunction with analgesic medications.

Muscle relaxants are divided into two categories: antispasmodic and antispasticity medications. Antispasmodics are used to treat muscle spasm resulting from injury, whereas antispasticity drugs are used

to treat patients with conditions such as cerebral palsy and spinal cord injuries. Our focus will be on the antispasmodics. You must always consider the potentially sedating effects of all muscle relaxants when they are prescribed. Thus, athletes must be warned about drowsiness that may interfere with attending classes, going to work, and participating in their sport.

Caution must also be used when combining muscle relaxants with narcotic analgesics; this can result in an additive effect and, consequently, increased sedation. Alcohol also has an additive effect that can increase sedation. Thus, given their limited efficacy and potential for sedation, muscle relaxants should be prescribed sparingly, if at all, in the athletic population. The following list represents the currently available muscle relaxants (all are administered orally and require a prescription):

- Carisoprodol (Soma)
- Chlorzoxazone (Paraflex, Parafon Forte)
- Cyclobenzaprine (Flexeril)
- Metaxalone (Skelaxin)
- Methocarbamol (Robaxin)
- Orphenadrine citrate (Antiflex, Norflex)

Guidelines for the Athletic Trainer

- Caution your athletes to never take the safety of any drug for granted, even one that is considered as safe as over-the-counter acetaminophen. Serious toxicity can result from overdoses of this seemingly innocuous substance. Advise athletes to never exceed the recommended dose of acetaminophen, particularly if they consume alcohol or do not eat regularly.

- Discourage your athletes from using combination drugs that contain caffeine. Research has shown that caffeine improves the effectiveness of analgesics (it is an ingredient in over-the-counter painkillers such as Anacin and Excedrin). However, in some individuals, even a modest dose could be enough to push the athlete's caffeine level above the acceptable limits of the NCAA or USOC, particularly if he or she has also consumed several servings of coffee, tea, or cola.[2] In most individuals, it takes about 1,000 mg of caffeine (8 cups of coffee) to result in a positive drug screen based on NCAA and IOC limits. Still, metabolism of caffeine varies among individuals, so a lower dose could result in a positive drug test.

- Discourage athletes from consuming alcohol in combination with any analgesic. The reasons for this vary for each specific drug, but the combination of ethanol and analgesics is detrimental in every instance.

- Make sure that athletes know that using painkillers to offset pain experienced during sport and exercise is not a wise course of action. Teach athletes that analgesics attack the symptom—pain—but do not treat the underlying cause. Masking the pain with a drug may cause a false sense of security and result in additional injury. The traditional RICE (rest, ice, compression, and elevation) approach for the treatment of sport injuries is often a better strategy.

- Ensure that caution is exercised in the use of opiate agonists, because the risk of developing a physical or psychological dependency (or both) is always a concern with these drugs.

References and Resources

1. Burger, A. 1986. *Drugs and people: Medications, their history and origins, and the way they act.* Charlottesville, VA: University Press of Virginia.

2. Fuentes, R.J., J.M. Rosenberg, and A. Davis. 1996. *Athletic drug reference '96.* Research Triangle Park, NC: Clean Data.

3. Luo, X., R. Pietrobon, L.H. Curtis, and L.A. Hey. 2004. Prescription of nonsteroidal anti-inflammatory drugs and muscle relaxants for back pain in the United States. *Spine* 29(23) (December):E531-E537.

4. National Collegiate Athletic Association. NCAA banned drug classes. www1.ncaa.org/membership/ed_outreach/health-safety/drug_testing/banned_drug_classes.pdf. Accessed 10/14/06.

5. Ortho-McNeil Pharmaceutical. 1996. Dear health care professional. Letter from the author, March 20, 1996.

6. Strom, B.L. 1994. Adverse reactions to over-the-counter analgesics taken for therapeutic purposes. *Journal of the American Medical Association (JAMA)* 272(23):1865-1867.

7. Time-Life Books, eds. 1996. *The medical advisor: The complete guide to alternative and conventional treatments.* Alexandria, VA: Time-Life.

8. Tramadol/Ultram. 1996. *Clinical pharmacology: An electronic drug reference and teaching guide.* Version 1.6. Gainesville, FL: Gold Standard Multimedia.

9. World Anti-Doping Agency. The world anti-doping code: The 2006 prohibited list. www.wada-ama.org/rtecontent/document/2006_LIST.pdf. Accessed 10/14/06.

10. Whitcomb, D.C., and G.D. Block. 1994. Association of acetaminophen hepatotoxicity with fasting and ethanol use. *Journal of the American Medical Association* 272(23):1845-1850.

11. Zimmerman, D.R. 1992. *Zimmerman's guide to nonprescription drugs.* 2nd ed. Detroit: Gale Research.

CHAPTER 6

Local Anesthetics and Topical Agents for Minor Pain

The painkillers that practitioners typically use on athletes fall into two broad categories: local, injectable anesthetics and topical pain relievers. Injectable anesthetics are available only by prescription and must be administered by a licensed medical practitioner. Over-the-counter topical anesthetics are readily available in a variety of strengths and formulations. They can be applied on an as-needed basis by you or the athletes themselves.

All anesthetics, whether injected or topically applied, work via the same mechanism. They reversibly block the conduction of impulses along nerve pathways and other membranes that use sodium channels to generate an action potential.

Pain that originates in the skin and the tissue layers immediately beneath the skin's surface differs little from other pain. Skin pain responds more readily to topical anesthetics and topical analgesics—drugs that specifically block the nerve receptors for pain in the skin. And since pain and itching are produced by the same sensory nerve endings in the skin (weak stimulation of the nerve fibers causes itching; strong stimulation causes pain), products designed for topical pain relief may also relieve itching.

The broad classification of topically applied anesthetics and analgesics includes such products as liniments, lotions, rubs, and creams that are marketed as remedies for relieving the pain of simple backache, strains, bruises, and sprains.[4] Many of these topical preparations designed to relieve underlying aches and pains fall into the category of substances known as *counterirritants*.

KEY TERMS

counterirritant

infiltrative anesthesia

injectable anesthetics

topical analgesic

topical anesthetic

vasoconstrictor

vasodilation

Broadly defined, a counterirritant is an agent that causes irritation or mild inflammation of the skin, with the objective of relieving the pain of a deep-seated inflammatory process. These agents are formulated as a lotion, cream, or gel. A counterirritant mildly stimulates the nerve endings in the skin that respond to warmth, coolness, and pain, thus distracting the user from a more bothersome pain that is deep seated in the muscles or bones. For example, the tingling sensation of a counterirritant applied directly to the skin over the shoulder overrides the pain impulse from an underlying strained muscle or joint. The intensity of the individual's response to a counterirritant depends on the specific irritant used, its concentration, the solvent in which it is dissolved, and the duration of its contact with the skin.

Injectable
Local Anesthetics

The FDA generally classifies injectable local anesthetics by their duration: short acting (up to 1 hour), intermediate acting (2 to 4 hours), or long acting (up to 8 hours). A large number of injectable anesthetics are available, but the two most widely used are the intermediate-acting lidocaine (Xylocaine) and the longer-acting bupivacaine (Marcaine). These medications may be used to infiltrate the skin before suturing a laceration, to block sensation of a finger (digital block), or to provide pain relief when injected into a joint. Injectable local anesthetics are only available with a prescription and should only be administered by a licensed medical practitioner.

Lidocaine is sometimes combined with epinephrine, which may prolong lidocaine's effectiveness when used to infiltrate tissue. Since epinephrine is a potent vasoconstrictor, it causes the blood vessels to contract, which maintains the local anesthetic level in the tissue and also controls bleeding. Physicians often avoid using the combination product of lidocaine and epinephrine because of a theoretical concern about ischemia if the product is used on fingers and toes. In addition, epinephrine and many other vasoconstrictors are banned from use during sanctioned competition; therefore, you must be sure to check the ingredients in a local anesthetic before approving its administration to an athlete.

Indications and Uses

The only injectable local anesthetics you will routinely encounter as an athletic trainer are those used for infiltrative anesthesia. This type of anesthesia involves the subcutaneous injection of a local anesthetic to interfere with sensory nerve function in a limited area of soft tissue, thus numbing the affected area.

In sports medicine, a team physician may consider injectable anesthetics for short-term pain management of the following conditions:[3]

- Soft tissue injuries
- Hip pointers
- Acromioclavicular (AC) joint sprain
- Turf toe
- Nondisplaced rib fractures
- Reduction of phalangeal dislocations

Side Effects
and Adverse Reactions

Local injectable anesthetics are usually quite safe when used as directed. It generally takes large quantities of these drugs to produce adverse reactions. Side effects may include stimulation of the central nervous system (tremors and seizures), drowsiness, cardiac arrhythmias, hypotension (only in toxic doses), and hypersensitivity reactions.

Topical Medications

Topical anesthetics are easy to spot on pharmacy shelves. They generally contain the suffix *caine* or *amine* in their brand names. As a rule, anesthetics with the *caine* suffix tend to be stronger and provide faster relief, but they are also more toxic.[9] Topical products that are corticosteroids (hydrocortisone and hydrocortisone acetate) can be used to stop itching, but they do not relieve pain.

Many of the topical products available for treating minor pain or injury contain various combinations of active and inactive ingredients. Topical painkillers can be categorized by (1) their primary activity (local anesthetic, counterirritant, or combination product), (2) their active ingredient, and (3) their lowest to highest concentration, by brand name. You can use this strategy to first decide which active ingredient you want to use, then to determine an appropriate strength, formulation, and brand.

Indications and Uses

A variety of topical anesthetics are available over the counter. In general, topical anesthetics should be used for quick relief of muscle or joint pain or minor skin irritations. Topical anesthetics are not intended for long-term use; their labeling states that they should be used only for "temporary relief of minor aches and pains of muscles and joints."

Local Anesthetics

Products labeled as topical anesthetics generally act to block *all* sensations in the skin, thereby causing a temporary numbing effect.

- **Benzocaine.** A safe and effective remedy for pain and itch, benzocaine is relatively insoluble in water. Since very little of this substance can penetrate the skin to enter the bloodstream, it does not exert some of the serious side effects associated with other "caine" products. Benzocaine's activity occurs almost wholly within the skin and mucous membranes, where it blocks pain-conducting nerve endings and provides long-lasting relief. One application may quell pain and itch for 4 to 6 hours.[9]

- **Dibucaine.** This extremely potent and long-acting synthetic substance begins to relieve pain and itch in as little as 15 minutes. If formulated in a base that keeps it moist and in direct contact with the skin's surface, dibucaine may continue to provide relief for up to 4 hours. Because of its potency, only small amounts of dibucaine are needed to provide pain relief for an individual. Dibucaine is readily absorbed, so you should not apply it to large areas of the body or to badly bruised, raw, or blistered skin; this may potentially increase systemic absorption.[9]

- **Lidocaine.** Lidocaine is widely used and is very safe when used as directed—applied to small areas of wounded or itchy skin. It is especially effective in treating itchiness, irritation, and pain of the mucous membranes. But, beware, if applied in large amounts to wide areas of bruised or broken skin, lidocaine can cause seizures or cardiac arrhythmias. Furthermore, lidocaine should not be used on raw or blistered skin because this may also potentially increase systemic absorption.[9]

- **Pramoxine.** Pramoxine does not belong to the "caine" family of pain relievers and therefore appears to be essentially free of their systemic side effects. It may, however, irritate some mucous membranes. Pramoxine is contraindicated for the eyes, and it may irritate the skin, causing a rash. Pramoxine is most effective for use on broken skin.[9]

- **Tetracaine.** Tetracaine relieves itching and pain on both damaged and undamaged skin, and it numbs damaged skin. Like other "caine" drugs, tetracaine can cause seizures or cardiac arrhythmias if applied in large amounts to wide areas of injured skin and the athlete's body absorbs it. However, this risk is remote because tetracaine should only be applied to small areas of skin. Tetracaine is longer acting than benzocaine.[9]

- **Ethyl chloride and dichlorofluoromethane.** These products evaporate very rapidly, temporarily "freezing" the skin. The duration of action is quite fast—approximately 1 minute. Rethawing may be mildly painful. These products provide significant local anesthesia to decrease pain associated with intramuscular and subcutaneous injections.[5] They may also be used to temporarily provide pain relief following contusions (such as being struck by a baseball), but they are more effective when used as an adjunct to injections.

- **Trolamine salicylate.** The mechanism of action for this topical analgesic is similar to that of other salicylates such as aspirin. The body absorbs trolamine salicylate from the skin. For example, when trolamine salicylate is applied over the knee, salicylate concentrations in synovial (joint) fluid are roughly 60% of those attained after a 500 mg oral dose of aspirin. Salicylate concentrations in the blood, however, are negligible after using topical trolamine salicylate.[3]

Counterirritants

As stated previously, counterirritants mildly stimulate nerve endings in the skin that respond to pain, warmth, and coolness. For the irritant substance to reach these sensory nerves, the body must absorb it through the skin's protective outer layers. Penetration of the epidermis by the irritant is more easily accomplished when the irritant is dissolved in oil, water, or some other substance that is actively absorbed by the skin. Hence, manufacturers typically formulate counterirritants as lotions, ointments, gels, and creams.

- **Capsaicin.** A derivative of the cayenne pepper, capsaicin creates a warm—even burning—sensation on the skin. In addition to its local irritant effect, capsaicin also limits the activity of substance P in transmitting pain messages to the central nervous system.[1] Although products containing this substance may feel intolerably hot, they do not cause blistering or reddening of the skin, and physicians consider them safe for relief of transitory aches and pains. Manufacturers also market stronger formulations for relief of the severe pain of arthritis, diabetic neuropathy, and herpes zoster (shingles).[9]

- **Menthol.** When rubbed vigorously onto the skin, menthol produces a feeling of coolness, even though the skin temperature in the treated area is in all likelihood warmer than the surrounding skin surface. At relatively high concentrations of 1.25 to 16%, menthol is stimulating and mildly irritating to the skin. Manufacturers use it as an ingredient in liniments and rubs. When used in low concentrations of 0.1 to 1.0%, menthol—usually combined with camphor or other external analgesic ingredients—is a safe and effective means of relieving itching and pain. It will penetrate broken as well as injured skin to reach sensory nerve endings. Menthol has an extremely pungent odor, but the vapors appear to be more soothing than harmful.[6]

- **Methyl salicylate.** Sometimes called *wintergreen oil*, this sweet-smelling member of the aspirin family is one of the most widely used counterirritants. Although it is extremely toxic, manufacturers use methyl salicylate in very low concentrations as a flavoring agent in candy, chewing gum, cough drops, and toothpaste. Ingestion of more than small amounts (as little as 4 mL) can be lethal. Methyl salicylate is currently available in the United States only in combination with other products.

Combination Products

Manufacturers frequently use menthol in combination with methyl salicylate. The following products contain these two counterirritants, with or without additional ingredients:

- Banalg (various products)
- Ben-Gay (various products)
- Flexall Pain Relieving Gel
- Heet
- Icy Hot (various products)
- Mentholatum (various products)

Many more products (too numerous to list here) are available that use combinations of the ingredients already discussed. When in doubt about which product to choose, consult a physician or pharmacist. Be sure to read all label directions before applying any topical anesthetic or analgesic.

Side Effects and Adverse Reactions

Toxicity is minimal after topical administration of local anesthetics unless they are applied to large areas of denuded skin (the epithelium is removed). In such cases, the body can absorb significant amounts of the drug into the systemic circulation, causing the adverse reactions noted.

The most severe—though rare—adverse reaction to using topical anesthetics occurs when large amounts of some "caine" preparations are applied to large areas of bruised or otherwise damaged skin. In these instances, much of the drug will be absorbed into the body. This systemic absorption can cause life-threatening toxic reactions—including seizures and cardiac arrhythmias. These reactions are highly unlikely when the medications are used as directed on the label.

More common and less severe side effects of topical anesthetics can include rashes, hives, and other skin eruptions—the very symptoms these drugs are supposed to relieve. Reactions such as these are not serious and usually abate when use is discontinued. People who have known systemic allergies to food and other substances should be especially careful when using topical anesthetics because such people may be more sensitive to these substances.

The location of a rash or injury, as well as the general condition of the skin surrounding it, can influence the action of a topical anesthetic. Some drugs are more readily absorbed through thin skin such as that found around the eyes, nose, and mouth.

In general, the FDA considers external analgesics safe for use by adults.[9] However, you should always check the label for appropriate use. The safety and effectiveness of individual products are complicated by the form these products take. Most are formulated as creams, sprays, or lotions in combination with inactive ingredients that influence the active drug's ability to reach and remain in contact with the skin. The concentration of the active ingredient also varies from one product to another. Users may need to try several products on a trial-and-error basis to find the one that best suits their particular situation. See table 6.1 for a summary of the more common topical anesthetics and counterirritants.

Considerations Before Use

Products containing methyl salicylate should never be used in combination with a heating pad or occlusive (tightly bound) dressing. This combination causes vasodilation (expansion of blood vessels), which increases the systemic absorption of methyl salicylate and can result in necrosis (tissue death) of the skin and muscle as well as interstitial nephritis (a disease of the structural connective tissue of the kidney). For the same reasons, products containing methyl salicylate should not be applied before exercising in hot or humid conditions or immediately following exercise. The product should only be applied after the body has had an opportunity to cool down.[3]

Athletes who are allergic to aspirin should not use methyl salicylate or trolamine salicylate because the body can absorb the salicylate in either of these products. In seriously allergic individuals, the risk of an adverse reaction is not dose related; even a very small amount of topically applied salicylate can generate an allergic response.

Counterirritants are designed to stimulate nerve impulses, while local anesthetics are designed to suppress those impulses. Although it is not dan-

Table 6.1 Summary of Common Topical Anesthetics and Counterirritants

Topical anesthetics	Counterirritants
Benzocaine	6% cream: Lanacane 20% gel: Hurricaine 20% liquid: Hurricaine 20% ointment: Americaine 20% spray: Americaine, Hurricaine, Solarcaine
Dibucaine	1% ointment: Nupercainal
Lidocaine	0.5% cream, gel, or spray: Solarcaine Aloe Extra Burn Relief 2.5% ointment: Xylocaine
Pramoxine	1% cream: Proctozone-P 1% lotion: Prax
Tetracaine	0.5% ointment: Pontocaine 1% cream: Pontocaine
Ethyl chloride and dichlorofluoromethane	Aerosol spray: AeroFreeze
Trolamine salicylate	10% topical cream: Aspercreme, Mobisyl, Myoflex, Sportscreme 10% topical lotion: Sportscreme
Capsaicin	0.025% cream: Arthricare, Capzasin-P, Zostrix 0.075% cream: Zostrix HP 0.075% lotion: Capzasin HP
Menthol	1.27% liquid: Absorbine Jr. 2.5% gel: Ben-Gay Daytime Pain Relieving Gel 3% gel: Ben-Gay Sports and Exercise Rub, Vanishing Scent 4% gel: Mineral Ice 4% gel: Absorbine Power Gel 4% liquid: Absorbine Jr. Extra Strength 7% topical gel: Flexall 454 8% topical cream: Eucalyptamint Muscle Pain Relief 15% ointment: Eucalyptamint Ointment

gerous to combine the two, it would be illogical to do so.[3]

Varying degrees of solubility in water and body fluids may also determine a product's effectiveness. A compound that is insoluble in water may be relatively worthless when applied to unbroken skin, but this compound may be highly effective on broken skin since it can reach underlying nerve endings. For best results on intact skin, look for external analgesics that are fat soluble. They may be more readily absorbed.

Currently, the NCAA and WADA permit the use of all "caine" derivative local anesthetics for topical, infiltrative, or intra-articular injection when medically justified. Intravenous injection of local anesthetics is banned by the NCAA[6] but is not specifically prohibited by WADA.[8]

Regulations regarding medication often vary between the NCAA and WADA and are always subject to change. For a complete and updated list of banned substances, contact the appropriate governing body.[6,8]

Guidelines for the Athletic Trainer

• Before administering any of the products discussed in this chapter, be sure to ask the athlete if he or she is allergic to aspirin or any local anesthetics.

• None of the topical painkillers described in this chapter is currently banned for use *before* competition. However, keep in mind that using these products before competition to offset exercise-limiting or incapacitating pain is inappropriate and could result in further injury to the athlete. Encourage the athlete to rest the injured area instead.

- Similarly, using these products week after week is ill-advised (although not necessarily toxic). Generally, an individual should not use these products for more than 7 consecutive days. You or the athlete should consult a physician for pain that persists beyond 1 week.[3]

- As with any seemingly harmless product, serious problems, even toxicity, can arise if a product is used inappropriately. Read and follow all instructions on labels. Expiration dates for creams and ointments are stamped on the crimped (folded) end of the tube; do not use a product beyond its expiration date.

- Avoid vigorous massage to an area after the application of a topical anesthetic. Massage causes cutaneous vasodilation, which may increase the possibility of systemic absorption.

- Absorption occurs more rapidly if the protective outer layers of the skin have been broken or scraped. To prevent possible damage to underlying tissues, avoid using topical pain relievers, especially counterirritants, on injured skin.

- Advise athletes on all of these precautions, because many athletes are likely to use these products without giving them a second thought.

References and Resources

1. Caterina, M.J., and D. Julius. 2001. The vanilloid receptor: A molecular gateway to the pain pathway. *Annu Rev Neurosci* 24:487-517.

2. *Clinical pharmacology: An electronic drug reference and teaching guide.* 1996. Version 1.6. Gainesville, FL: Gold Standard Multimedia.

3. Covington, T.R., R.R. Berardi, and L.L. Young, eds. 1993. *Handbook of nonprescription drugs.* 10th ed. Washington, D.C.: American Pharmaceutical Association.

4. Fuentes, R.J., J.M. Rosenberg, and A. Davis. 1996. *Athletic drug reference '96.* Research Triangle Park, NC: Clean Data.

5. Mawhorter, S., L. Daugherty, A. Ford, R. Hughes, D. Metzger, and K. Easley. 2004. Topical vapocoolant quickly and effectively reduces vaccine-associated pain: Results of a randomized, single-blinded, placebo-controlled study. *Journal of Travel Medicine* 11(5) (September):267-272.

6. National Collegiate Athletic Association. NCAA banned drug classes. www1.ncaa.org/membership/ed_outreach/health-safety/drug_testing/banned_drug_classes.pdf. Accessed 10/14/06.

7. Time-Life Books, eds. 1996. *The medical advisor: The complete guide to alternative and conventional treatments.* Alexandria, VA: Time-Life.

8. World Anti-Doping Agency. The world anti-doping code: The 2006 prohibited list. www.wada-ama.org/rtecontent/document/2006_LIST.pdf. Accessed 10/14/06.

9. Zimmerman, D.R. 1992. *Zimmerman's guide to nonprescription drugs.* 2nd ed. Detroit: Gale Research.

CHAPTER 7

Systemic Drugs Used to Treat Infections

After musculoskeletal injuries, infectious diseases will likely be the most common malady you encounter in your athletes. Ranging from strep throat to ringworm, many of these infections will require treatment with a systemic anti-infective medication. In this chapter we will discuss the three classes of systemic medications used to fight infections: antibiotics, antifungals, and antivirals.

Antibiotic Medications

Antibiotics are used to fight bacterial infections. Bacterial infections are by far the most common indication for the use of systemic anti-infectives, and multiple classifications of antibiotics are used to treat numerous infections.

Indications and Uses

When physicians prescribe an antibiotic to treat an infection, they must consider what specific bacterium is most likely to be the invading organism. In some cases, such as skin infections producing pus, bacterial cultures can be obtained, and the pathogen can be isolated and identified. This is also the case for urinary tract infections. Sensitivity testing may then determine which antibiotics will be most effective in treating the infection. However, this process may take several days, and antibiotic treatment must be started before receiving the test results. Thus, the physician uses his or her experience to determine which antibiotic is *most likely* to be effective.

> **KEY TERMS**
>
> broad-spectrum antibiotic
> cephalosporins
> floroquinolones
> influenza
> macrolides
> narrow-spectrum antibiotic
> penicillins

In most cases, an antibiotic that primarily affects the targeted bacteria should be used. This is what is called a *narrow-spectrum antibiotic.* Using a narrow-spectrum antibiotic limits side effects (those side effects caused by the destruction of beneficial bacteria in the gastrointestinal tract or vagina) and prevents the development of antibiotic resistance. Thus, if an athlete has strep throat and no allergies to penicillin, penicillin should be used because it has the narrowest spectrum of activity. A medication in the floroquinolone class would also be effective, but those medications have a *broad spectrum* of activity and would destroy other bacteria throughout the body. Any time bacteria are exposed to an antibiotic, there is a risk of causing resistant strains of bacteria.

Antibiotics are used for an array of illnesses. In a young athletic population, you will likely encounter athletes using antibiotics for the prophylactic

45

treatment of acne. The tetracyclines are most commonly used for this purpose. The most common illnesses requiring antibiotic treatment are those of the respiratory system, including strep throat, sinusitis, and pneumonia. Athletes must be reminded that upper-respiratory infections and bronchitis are often viral and will not respond to antibiotic treatment. Thus, an athlete should not expect to receive antibiotics from a physician for treatment of the common cold.

Sexually transmitted diseases are not uncommon in young adults, so you will likely encounter athletes being treated for such conditions. Since compliance with a medication treatment regimen is always difficult, it is fortunate that gonorrhea (treated with oral cefixime or intramuscular ceftriaxone) and chlamydia (treated with azithromycin) infections are both cured with a single dose of the appropriate antibiotic.

Distinguishing Features

Multiple classes of antibiotics are available for physicians to choose from when prescribing a medication to fight a particular infection. The following sections outline the basic features that distinguish one class of antibiotics from another.

Penicillin

Penicillin was discovered in 1928 but did not come into widespread use until the 1940s. It effectively inhibits the synthesis of bacterial cell walls by attaching to specific enzymes that are responsible for cell wall construction. Therefore, the bacterium is unable to maintain its cell wall stability and is destroyed. Human cells do not have a wall and are unaffected by the medication.

Penicillin and its derivatives all contain the same basic chemical structure, a beta-lactam ring (see figure 7.1). This ring is essential to penicillin's antibacterial activity. Certain bacteria are capable of producing an enzyme called *beta-lactamase*, which destroys the beta-lactam ring. If the beta-lactam ring is destroyed, the drug becomes ineffective. This is the way that many bacteria acquire resistance to penicillin and its derivatives.

The terms *gram-positive* and *gram-negative* are used to describe a bacterial organism's penchant for absorbing a dye called "Gram's stain" that colors the organism purple and renders it visible under a microscope. Organisms that absorb the dye and appear purple under magnification are gram-positive; gram-negative organisms are those that absorb little or none of the dye and appear faint pink under the microscope.

The penicillin family is most effective against gram-positive bacteria. Gram-positive bacteria are often responsible for skin infections and respiratory infections. Unfortunately, many of these bacteria have developed resistance to penicillin over the years. *Streptococcus pyogenes,* the bacterium responsible for strep throat, remains very sensitive to penicillin. However, *Streptococcus pneumoniae* and several *Staphylococcus* species are resistant.

A specific type of bacteria, methicillin-resistant *Staphylococcus aureus* (MRSA), has received a great deal of attention in both the lay and medical press. This bacterial strain has been responsible for a number of outbreaks of cellulitis and boils across the country, both in hospitals and among athletic teams.[2] MRSA can be easily spread by asymptomatic carriers and may cause serious infections that are difficult to treat. Any athlete with a suspected MRSA infection should have the infected wound examined by a physician; cultures of the wound must be obtained to determine the specific bacterium causing the infection and to discover what antibiotics will be effective against it.

Although not effective against MRSA, one specific defense against beta-lactamase has been developed. Clavulanic acid acts as a competitive inhibitor of beta-lactamase, inhibiting the action of the enzyme on the beta-lactam ring of the accompanying antibiotic. Clavulanic acid is combined with amoxicillin in an oral form (Augmentin) and with ticarcillin in an intravenous form (Timentin).

Cephalosporins

Cephalosporins have a similar structure and mechanism of action to the penicillins. The cephalosporins have been classified into four generations as newer agents have been developed over the years. The first generation is most effective against gram-positive

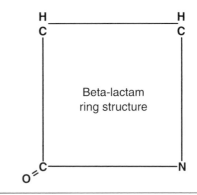

Figure 7.1 The beta-lactam ring structure that is essential to the function of the penicillin family.

bacteria. Each subsequent generation has been developed to have increasing effectiveness against gram-negative bacteria (e.g., E. coli, salmonella), with some of the agents maintaining efficacy against the gram-positive bacteria.

Sulfonamides

Sulfonamides were widely used even before penicillin, but they are not as effective as the penicillins for most infections. For example, they are completely ineffective against strep throat. "Sulfa drugs" act against invading bacteria by inhibiting the bacteria's ability to synthesize folic acid. These drugs are particularly effective in treating most urinary tract infections. They have also come back into wider use in treating skin infections because they are effective against most strains of MRSA. The sulfonamide sulfamethoxazole is most commonly used in combination with trimethoprim, an antibiotic that acts by interfering with the action of bacteria, inhibiting synthesis of tetrahydrofolic acid. Tetrahydrofolic acid is an essential precursor in the DNA components of bacteria.

Tetracyclines

Tetracyclines have a broad spectrum of activity against a variety of bacteria. They inhibit bacterial protein synthesis. Tetracyclines are most commonly used for the treatment of acne because they are well tolerated and they are effective against the bacteria that cause acne. Minocycline is the most common tetracycline used for this indication. Although these drugs are easily absorbed following ingestion, foods or products containing calcium, magnesium, iron, aluminum, or zinc will impair the absorption of the tetracyclines.

Macrolides

Macrolides also inhibit bacterial protein synthesis. This class of antibiotics has a similar spectrum of activity to the penicillins and can be used in individuals with a penicillin allergy. They are commonly used in the treatment of respiratory infections, such as sinusitis, strep throat, and pneumonia. The frequently used agents include erythromycin, azithromycin (Zithromax), and clarithromycin (Biaxin). Azithromycin has become very popular because it has limited GI side effects and once-a-day dosing.

Aminoglycosides

Aminoglycosides are primarily available for intravenous use, except for the topically applied neomycin and an inhaled formulation of tobramycin (used for individuals with cystic fibrosis). These agents inhibit bacterial protein synthesis and are very effective against gram-negative bacteria.

Floroquinolones

Floroquinolones have become very popular over the past decade because they have a broad spectrum of activity, few side effects, and once- or twice-a-day dosing. They exert their effect by interfering with the coiling process of bacterial DNA. These drugs are widely used for the treatment of pneumonia and urinary tract infections.

Routes of Administration

If a person is severely ill—and is unable to take or keep down antibiotics because of nausea and vomiting—or a person is at risk for dehydration, then intravenous administration of the medication is indicated. Intravenous delivery of most antibiotics results in a higher concentration of the medication in the bloodstream. As the infection resolves, the individual can typically switch over to an oral medication. In rare cases, such as with an infected bone or joint, intravenous antibiotic courses of up to 6 weeks in duration may be indicated. In these instances, special catheters can be placed in the veins, and the antibiotics can be given once or twice daily at home.

In some instances, intramuscular administration of an antibiotic is indicated. This is typically in cases where one injection can eliminate the need for 7 to 10 days of oral antibiotics. Strep throat is a good example of this; however, a single injection of penicillin is not always as effective as a course of oral antibiotics. Intramuscular injection of ceftriaxone for a gonorrhea infection is occasionally used to ensure that the infected individual is properly treated.

Side Effects and Adverse Reactions

All antibiotics can cause nausea, vomiting, and diarrhea. Erythromycin tends to be tolerated less well than other medications. The use of penicillin can result in an allergic reaction ranging from a mild rash to anaphylaxis. Individuals who have developed a rash in response to penicillin can safely use a cephalosporin because the risk of cross-reactivity is less than 10%. Such a risk is not acceptable for a person with a history of anaphylaxis.

Although typically well tolerated, the "sulfa" medications can cause a rare—but potentially fatal—cutaneous reaction called *Stevens-Johnson syndrome*. Anyone developing a rash while taking a sulfa drug should be evaluated by a physician. Though you will rarely encounter the use of aminoglycosides, you should be aware that toxic levels of these drugs in the blood may result in hearing loss, so blood levels must be carefully monitored when these drugs are used.

The tetracyclines can also cause gastrointestinal distress, but the symptoms can be alleviated if the medication is taken with food. A more concerning effect of the tetracyclines is that they increase the skin's sensitivity to ultraviolet light. This photosensitivity reaction may result in exaggerated sunburns following even moderate exposure to the sun when taking these medications.

A *bacterial infection* is defined as a detrimental colonization of a host organism by a foreign species.[5] The infecting organism, or pathogen, interferes with the normal functioning of the host. Several systems of the body normally function with a beneficial bacterial colonization. In many instances, the use of antibiotics to fight a pathogenic bacterial infection may also disrupt the balance of beneficial bacteria in the body. Side effects from this may include the development of vaginal yeast infections or a severe form of diarrhea resulting from an overabundance of the bacterium *Clostridium difficile* in the colon. These infections result from a disruption of normal bacterial flora within the vagina and colon, respectively.

Table 7.1 provides a summary of antibiotic medications, including their mode of action, indications, and side effects or adverse reactions.

Antifungal Medications

Antifungals are used to fight fungal infections. They are most commonly used in their topical form, but the type of infection will determine the route of administration for the medication. Many of the antifungal medications are available in oral, intravenous, and topical forms. (See chapter 8 for more information on topical antifungals.)

Indications and Uses

Most fungal infections that affect athletes are cured through the use of topical medications (see chapter 8). However, certain infections will best respond to oral medications. Multiple fungal lesions of the skin (tinea corporis) may be more easily eradicated with oral medications than with topical applications. Infections involving the scalp (tinea capitis),

other hair follicles, or the nail beds (onchmycosis) must be treated orally to allow the medication to be incorporated into the hair shaft, or nail bed, to kill the invading fungus. The treatment of vaginal yeast infections can be conveniently accomplished with a single dose of oral fluconazole. Many antifungal medications are also available for intravenous use.

Distinguishing Features

The oral antifungal agents act to impair the biosynthesis of ergosterol, a component of the fungal cell membrane. The currently available agents all share many similarities. Ketoconazole is inexpensive but is being less commonly used because of its potential for hepatotoxicity (liver damage). Traconazole has been replacing ketoconazole for use in treating a variety of infections. The most common indications for the use of traconazole in athletes are tinea corporis and vaginal yeast infections. Fluconazole is available in a single dose for the treatment of vaginal yeast infections and is also effective against ringworm. Griseofulvin is deposited in keratin cells and is therefore highly effective in the treatment of fungal infections involving the scalp. In order to completely eradicate the infection from the keratin cells, treatment may last up to 2 months.

Routes of Administration

As previously discussed, several antifungal medications are available in topical, oral, and intravenous formulations. Systemic fungal infections requiring intravenous medication are most commonly encountered in severely immunocompromised individuals, and the treatment of these infections is beyond the scope of this discussion.

Side Effects and Adverse Reactions

Similar to antibiotics, antifungal medication may cause gastrointestinal irritation. The biggest concern with the antifungal medications is their interaction with other medications. Antifungals can potentially increase or decrease the plasma levels of multiple agents, including antibiotics, proton pump inhibitors, and antiepileptic drugs. If an athlete has been given a prescription for an antifungal, the athlete must let the pharmacist know if he or she is already taking any other medications.

Table 7.2 provides a summary of antifungal medications, including their mode of action, indications, and side effects or adverse reactions.

Table 7.1 Antibiotic Medications

Classification	Mode of action	Indications	Side effects and adverse reactions

Penicillins
Penicillin VK
Aminopenicillins
Ampicillin (Omnipen)
Amoxicillin (Amoxil)
Amoxicillin
  with clavulanic acid
  (Augmentin)
	Inhibits the synthesis of bacterial cell walls by attaching to specific enzymes that are responsible for cell wall construction	Gram-positive bacterial skin infections
		Gram-positive respiratory infections
			• Nausea
			• Vomiting
			• Diarrhea
			• Allergic reaction
			• Vaginal yeast infections
			• Skin rash

Cephalosporins
First generation
  Cephalexin (Keflex)
  Cefadroxil (Duricef)
	Same as penicillins	Gram-positive bacteria	• Nausea
			• Vomiting
			• Diarrhea
			• Vaginal yeast infections

Second generation
  Cefprozil (Cefzil)
  Cefaclor (Ceclor)
  Cefpodoxime (Vantin)
  Cefdinir (Omnicef)
		Skin infections
		Ear infections
			• Nausea
			• Vomiting
			• Diarrhea
			• Vaginal yeast infections

Third generation
  Cefixime (Suprax)
  Ceftriaxone* (Rocephin)
		Gonorrhea	• Nausea
			• Vomiting
			• Diarrhea
			• Vaginal yeast infections

Aminoglycosides Tobramycin Gentamicin* Amikacin (Amikin)	Inhibits bacterial protein synthesis	Gram-negative bacteria	• Nausea • Vomiting • Diarrhea • Vaginal yeast infections • Nephrotoxicity

Sulfonamide
Sulfamethoxazole
  with trimethoprim
  (Bactrim, Septra)
	Inhibits bacteria's ability to synthesize folic acid	Urinary tract infections
		Skin infections such as MRSA
			• Nausea
			• Vomiting
			• Diarrhea
			• Skin rash
			• Stevens-Johnson syndrome (rare, but potentially fatal, cutaneous reaction)

Floroquinolones Ciprofloxacin (Cipro) Levofloxacin (Levaquin) Gatifloxacin (Tequin) Moxifloxacin (Avelox)	Interferes with the coiling process of bacterial DNA	Pneumonia Urinary tract infections	• Nausea • Vomiting • Diarrhea
Macrolides Erythromycin Azithromycin (Zithromax) Clarithromycin (Biaxin)	Inhibits bacterial protein synthesis	Sinusitis Strep throat Pneumonia	• Nausea • Vomiting • Diarrhea
Tetracyclines Minocycline (Minocin) Doxycycline Tetracycline	Inhibits bacterial protein synthesis	Acne Respiratory infections	• Nausea† • Vomiting† • Diarrhea† • Increased photosensitivity

*intravenous or intramuscular administration only
†can be minimized by taking with food

Table 7.2 Antifungal Medications

Classification	Mode of action	Indications	Side effects and adverse reactions
Terbinafine (Lamisil)	Impairs biosynthesis of cell wall	Fungal infections of fingernails and toenails	• Gastrointestinal irritation • Can potentially increase or decrease the plasma levels of multiple agents, including antibiotics, proton pump inhibitors, and antiepileptic drugs
Ketoconazole (Nizoral)	Impairs biosynthesis of cell wall	Candidal infections of skin and mouth Tinea infections of skin	• Gastrointestinal irritation • Can potentially increase or decrease the plasma levels of multiple agents, including antibiotics, proton pump inhibitors, and antiepileptic drugs • Potential to cause hepatotoxicity
Itraconazole (Sporanox)	Impairs biosynthesis of cell wall	Tinea corporis Vaginal yeast infections Fungal infections of fingernails and toenails	• Gastrointestinal irritation • Can potentially increase or decrease the plasma levels of multiple agents, including antibiotics, proton pump inhibitors, and antiepileptic drugs
Fluconazole (Diflucan)	Impairs biosynthesis of cell wall	Vaginal yeast infections Ringworm	• Gastrointestinal irritation • Can potentially increase or decrease the plasma levels of multiple agents, including antibiotics, proton pump inhibitors, and antiepileptic drugs
Griseofulvin	Impairs biosynthesis of cell wall	Fungal infections involving the scalp	• Gastrointestinal irritation • Can potentially increase or decrease the plasma levels of multiple agents, including antibiotics, proton pump inhibitors, and antiepileptic drugs

Antiviral Medications

Antivirals are infrequently used in a healthy, athletic population because few common viral infections (such as upper-respiratory infections) respond to antiviral medications. In recent years, however, we have seen a rise in the use of antiviral medications in athletes, including for the treatment of influenza and the prevention of herpes infections in wrestlers.

Indications and Uses

The indications for the use of antiviral medications in an otherwise healthy athlete are limited. The medications used to treat influenza are further discussed later in this chapter. The primary varicella infection (chicken pox) is now rare because of the use of vaccinations, but when it does occur, acyclovir is effective in shortening the duration of symptoms if started within 24 hours of the onset of rash. Antiviral medications are also effective in treating herpes zoster (shingles), both for shortening the duration of the lesions and limiting the severity of pain following the resolution of the lesions.

In athletics, antiviral medications may be most commonly used in the treatment and prevention of lesions caused by the herpes simplex virus (HSV) in wrestlers (*Herpes gladiatorum*). The occurrence of HSV lesions during a wrestler's season can be devastating. Evidence suggests that the use of valacyclovir may prevent the reoccurrence of HSV lesions following a primary infection.[1]

Distinguishing Features

The medications commonly used for the treatment of viral infections in athletes act by interfering with the virus' ability to synthesize DNA. Acyclovir and valacyclovir are similar in structure and activity. Both have similar results against HSV, but valacyclovir is superior in treating herpes zoster. Famciclovir has a slightly different chemical structure but a similar spectrum of activity.

Many other antiviral medications are in use, including those used to treat influenza. Other targeted infections include hepatitis viruses, cytomegalovirus, and HIV. A full discussion of the broad array of antiviral drugs is beyond the scope of this text.

Influenza is prevalent in the United States in the late fall, winter, and early spring. Classic flu illness is characterized by the abrupt onset of fever (100-104 °F; 38-40 °C), chills, cough, rhinorrhea, sore throat, malaise, myalgias, headache, and anorexia.[3] In the athletic setting, early diagnosis and treatment of influenza can both limit the effects of the disease in the afflicted athlete and limit transmission to teammates. Thus, any athlete suspected of having influenza should be evaluated by the team physician as soon as possible.

The influenza virus belongs to the *Orthomyxoviridae* family. Three types of influenza viruses exist: A, B, and C. Only A and B are associated with human epidemics. The virus is spread via small, aerosolized particles or direct contact with respiratory secretions and is primarily spread through person-to-person contact.

Four anti-influenza drugs are currently available: amantadine (Symmetrel), rimantadine (Flumadine), oseltamivir (Tamiflu), and zanamivir (Relenza). When initiated within the first 48 hours of illness, these medications may decrease fever, decrease the severity of other symptoms, and reduce the duration of the illness by 1 to 1 1/2 days.[3] Treatment may also decrease the spread of the virus to others. Amantadine and rimantadine are only effective against influenza A. They work by blocking the function of a channel protein needed for viral replication. Both drugs are administered orally. Oseltamivir and zanamivir are neuraminidase inhibitors and are effective against influenza A and B. Neuraminidase inhibitors block the enzyme's activity and inhibit new virus particles from being released from the infected cell—thus limiting the spread of infection. Zanamivir is available as an orally inhaled powder. Oseltamivir is administered orally.

Routes of Administration

As previously described, antiviral medications are available in topical, oral, intravenous, and inhaled formulations. As with the antifungal and antibiotic medications, the type of infection dictates the route of administration. The use of intravenous antiviral medications in otherwise healthy young athletes is uncommon.

Side Effects and Adverse Reactions

The antiviral medications are generally well tolerated, but they may cause diarrhea, nausea, or vomiting. Oral acyclovir may cause a rash. Intravenous acyclovir has resulted in kidney damage.

Amantadine (Symmetrel), used for treating influenza A, has been associated with adverse neurological effects such as insomnia, anxiety, and depression in about 10 to 15% of patients, mainly in those with impaired renal function.[3] Rimantadine, also an anti-influenza drug used to treat influenza A, causes side effects in the central nervous system in about 2% of users. Both drugs may cause mild gastrointestinal symptoms. Resistance to amantadine and rimantadine develops rapidly in 25 to 35% of treated individuals.[3]

Zanamivir (the anti-influenza drug used to treat influenza A and B) has few side effects, although bronchospasm has been reported in persons with underlying lung diseases such as asthma.[4] The most common side effects associated with oseltamivir, another drug used to treat influenza A and B, are nausea and vomiting (in about 10 to 20% of users).[3] Resistance to both of these medications has been reported but is not as common as with the amantadines.[4]

Table 7.3 provides a summary of antiviral medications, including their mode of action, indications, and side effects or adverse reactions.

Considerations Before Use

A physician must consider several factors when prescribing medications for an infectious process. Foremost among these considerations is the type of infection being treated. As discussed, some antibiotics are superior to others in the treatment of specific conditions or organisms. For example, penicillin is nearly 100% effective in the treatment of strep throat, but it is ineffective in treating most skin infections. Thus, physicians will prescribe certain classifications of medications for specific conditions.

The second consideration must be whether the athlete has any specific drug allergies or has poorly tolerated a medicine in the past. An athlete who has had an allergic reaction to penicillin (or a penicillin derivative) in the past is certain to have another reaction if given another member of the penicillin family. If the reaction was a rash, the athlete

Table 7.3   Antiviral Medications

Classification	Mode of action	Indications	Side effects and adverse reactions
Valacyclovir (Valtrex)	Interferes with the virus' ability to synthesize DNA	Herpes simplex virus (HSV)	• Nausea • Diarrhea • Vomiting
Acyclovir (Zovirax)	Interferes with the virus' ability to synthesize DNA	Chicken pox HSV Herpes zoster	• Nausea • Diarrhea • Vomiting • Rash • Nephrotoxicity (IV only)
Famciclovir (Famvir)	Interferes with the virus' ability to synthesize DNA	HSV Herpes zoster	• Nausea • Diarrhea • Vomiting
Anti-influenza Amantadine (Symmetrel)	Blocks the function of a channel protein needed for viral replication	Influenza A	• Insomnia, anxiety, and depression (in 10-15% of patients, especially in those with impaired renal function) • Mild gastrointestinal symptoms
Rimantadine (Flumadine)	Blocks the function of a channel protein needed for viral replication	Influenza A	• Side effects in the central nervous system (in 2% of users) • Mild gastrointestinal symptoms
Oseltamivir (Tamiflu)	Acts as a neuraminidase inhibitor	Influenza A and B	• Nausea and vomiting (in about 10-20% of users)
Zanamivir (Relenza)	Acts as a neuraminidase inhibitor	Influenza A and B	• Bronchospasm has been reported in individuals with underlying lung diseases such as asthma

can safely be given a cephalosporin. However, if an athlete has ever had an anaphylactic reaction to penicillin, he or she should not be given any penicillin derivatives or members of the cephalosporin family.

As with any other medication, if there are questions regarding the athlete's compliance with taking the prescribed medication, two important factors must be considered: side effects and dosing schedule. As the symptoms of an infection begin to resolve, the occurrence of any side effect will provide a convenient excuse for the athlete to discontinue the use of a medication. Dosing schedule is important because a medication is more likely to be taken as prescribed if it needs to be taken only once or twice per day. Individuals are less likely to adhere to medication courses requiring three or more daily doses. Erythromycin provides an excellent example of both points. Although this drug is inexpensive and is very effective for a variety of infections, it frequently causes gastrointestinal distress and requires three or four daily doses.

Other than the potential problems discussed under "Side Effects and Adverse Reactions," none of the medications discussed in this chapter has any known negative effects on athletic performance. In fact, because all these medications are primarily focused on treating an infective illness, their proper and timely administration should allow the athlete to perform at his or her standard level following the resolution of the infection and its symptoms.

Currently, the NCAA and WADA permit the use of all classes of antibiotics discussed in this chapter. Regulations regarding medication often vary between the NCAA[6] and WADA[7] and are always subject to change. For a complete and updated list of banned substances, contact the appropriate governing body.

Guidelines for the Athletic Trainer

The role of the athletic trainer in the treatment of infectious diseases requiring systemic medication is multifaceted. Although you cannot prescribe the medications, you are in the position to identify the athletes who require such treatment. Thus, athletes showing systemic signs of illness (fever, vomiting, malaise) or athletes with worsening skin infections (bacterial, viral, or fungal) should be promptly referred to a physician. In addition, in cases where athletes have simple upper-respiratory infections (afebrile, sore throat, runny nose), you can reinforce the message that no anti-infective medications are needed.

Athletic trainers normally have more frequent contact with athletes than most physicians do; therefore, the athletic trainer is in a unique position to both monitor and encourage compliance with any prescribed medication regimens. This includes reminding athletes that even though they may feel better, they should continue to take the medication according to their physicians' instructions. You can help prevent the troublesome situation where individuals fail to complete a course of medication and then self-administer the remaining pills the next time they develop symptoms of illness. You are also in the position to monitor the occurrence of any allergic reactions or adverse effects.

References and Resources

1. Anderson, B.J. 1999. The effectiveness of valacyclovir in preventing reactivation of herpes gladiatorum in wrestlers. *Clin J Sport Med* 9(2) (April):86-90.

2. U.S. Department of Health and Human Services, Centers for Disease Control and Prevention. Healthcare-associated methicillin resistant *Staphylococcus aureus* (HA-MRSA). www.cdc.gov/ncidod/dhqp/ar_mrsa.html. Accessed 11/18/06.

3. Cheung, M., and J.M. Lieberman. 2002. Influenza: Update on strategies for management. Part 1. *Contemp Pediatr* 19(10):82-94.

4. Centers for Disease Control and Prevention (CDC). 1999. Neuraminidase inhibitors for treatment of influenza A and B infections. *MMWR Morb Mortal Wkly Rep* 48;RR-14:1.

5. Wikipedia. Infection. www.en.wikipedia.org/wiki/Bacterial_infection. Accessed 11/18/06.

6. National Collegiate Athletic Association. NCAA banned drug classes. www1.ncaa.org/membership/ed_outreach/health-safety/drug_testing/banned_drug_classes.pdf. Accessed 10/14/06.

7. World Anti-Doping Agency. The world anti-doping code: The 2006 prohibited list. www.wada-ama.org/rtecontent/document/2006_LIST.pdf. Accessed 10/14/06.

CHAPTER 8

Topical Preparations
Used to Treat or Prevent Infections

Topical preparations used on skin wounds and eruptions (referred to as anti-infectives) take one of three basic forms: antiseptics, antibiotics, or antifungals. Table 8.1 lists the indications for use and the possible side effects of the topical anti-infective medications that are most commonly used.

Antiseptics

Antiseptics are externally applied agents that stop the growth of microorganisms before they infect the individual. They are usually made from disinfectant chemicals that destroy bacteria on contact before these microorganisms have a chance to take hold in a wound. Examples of common antiseptics include plain rubbing alcohol (isopropanol) and tincture of iodine.

Indications and Uses

Over the past few years, a large increase has been seen in reports of serious skin infections in athletes.[2,5] Although many skin conditions are benign and will respond to a variety of over-the-counter treatments, you must suspect that every skin lesion is potentially contagious and dangerous. Because of the nature of their sport, wrestlers are at the greatest risk for contracting and spreading fungal, bacterial, and viral infections. The infectious agent that is potentially the most serious is community-acquired, methicillin-resistant *Staphylococcus aureus* (MRSA). This bacterium is resistant to a variety of medications and may result in cellulitis and the formation of abscesses.

KEY TERMS

antiseptics
athlete's foot
candidiasis
dermatophytid reaction
gram-negative bacteria
gram-positive bacteria
jock itch
MRSA
ringworm
shingles
tetanus

You may use both antiseptics and antibiotics to prevent infection in minor cuts, wounds, and abrasions. Furthermore, you may use antibiotics to treat superficial skin infections caused by microorganisms that are susceptible to these medications. Antifungals are effective only for the treatment of infections caused by fungal molds or yeasts (see sidebar on page 56).

As a general rule, topical antiseptics are most appropriate for use on large, open skin wounds. However, you should take care to select non-irritating antiseptics for use on wide areas of abraded skin. Antiseptics are typically formulated as swab-on

Table 8.1 Common Indications and Possible Side Effects of Anti-Infective Medications

Medication	Use	Possible side effects
Antiseptics		
Acetic acid	Swimmer's ear	Burning, stinging
Alcohols	Skin cleanser	Irritation of open wounds
Chlorhexidine	Skin cleanser	Mild skin irritation
Hydrogen peroxide	Wound cleanser	Irritation of open wounds
Iodines	Skin cleanser	Skin irritation Allergic reaction
Antibiotics		
Bacitracin zinc	Gram-positive skin infections	Hypersensitivity Nephrotoxicity*
Neomycin	Gram-positive skin infections	Hypersensitivity Nephrotoxicity*
Polymyxin B sulfate	Gram-negative skin infections	Nephrotoxicity*
Antifungals		
Clotrimazole	Fungal and yeast infections	Mild skin irritation*
Miconazole nitrate	Fungal and yeast infections	Mild skin irritation*
Tolnaftate	Fungal infections	Mild skin irritation*

*very rare occurrence

Common Sites of Fungal and Yeast Infections

Athlete's foot (tinea pedis)

Jock itch (tinea cruris)

Body ringworm (tinea corporis)

Scalp ringworm (tinea capitis)

Nail ringworm (tinea unguium)

Candidal infections—vagina, vulva, groin, feet

liquids, sprays, powders, and moist paper wipes. Their primary purpose is to cleanse the skin of germs around splinters, cuts, scratches, abrasions, and other superficial wounds. They are for external use only.

General Dose Protocols

Before using a topical antiseptic or antibiotic, you should clean the affected area with mild soap and cool water, if possible. In the absence of water, plain rubbing alcohol (isopropanol) is an excellent cleanser, but it is quite irritating, so avoid using it on large areas of abraded skin.

Distinguishing Features

The following antiseptic products are widely available over the counter:

• **Acetic acid.** Used mainly in the ear, this clear organic acid with a distinctive pungent odor provides protection against *Pseudomonas*, the cause of swimmer's ear. Acetic acid is available in pharmacies as Vosol-HC (by prescription only), which includes hydrocortisone, and Star Otic (OTC), as well as in many generic formulations. The user may experience some mild burning or stinging in the ear canal for a few minutes following application.

• **Alcohols (isopropyl alcohol, ethyl alcohol).** Alcohol is an excellent antiseptic for cleansing the skin before an injection or before drawing blood, but it is not the best choice for use on broken skin because it is so irritating to tissue. Therefore, you should not use alcohols on large wounds, puncture wounds, burns, or deeply embedded splinters. On the positive side, alcohols loosen, dissolve, and remove grease, oil, dirt, and debris from skin. In addition, they evaporate quickly, and because they are colorless, they do not stain clothing or skin; therefore, they will not mask any changes in skin color around a wound that might indicate infection. Isopropyl alcohol (common rubbing alcohol; also called *isopropanol*) kills bacteria on contact, including *Staphylococcus aureus* and *Escherichia coli*. It is for external use only as an antiseptic or rub. The vapors from isopropyl alcohol are extremely toxic, so you should only use it as a rub in well-ventilated areas. Ethyl alcohol (the ingestible alcohol in liquor; also called *ethanol*) is a less effective bactericidal agent. It will kill some viruses but is largely ineffective against fungal cells. You should not use it on wide, open wounds because in large amounts, ethanol is quite irritating and may kill white blood cells.[8]

• **Chlorhexidine (Hibiclens).** Used primarily as a hand scrub in hospitals, chlorhexidine provides effective protection against *Staphylococcus* and some gram-negative bacteria. Chlorhexidine may also be helpful in treating individuals who develop frequent staphylococcus infections. Using chlorhexidine as a whole body cleanser with showering over a period of 2 weeks may decrease the number of bacteria colonized on a person's body, thus decreasing the risk for further skin infections. Chlorhexidine is not effective against the bacterial spores that cause tetanus.[3]

• **Hydrogen peroxide.** The foaming and bubbling action of this commonly used bactericide helps remove debris from wounds. To release oxygen and be effective, however, hydrogen peroxide must come into direct contact with blood or tissue fluids; therefore, it is ineffective on unbroken skin. Note, too, that no one should ever use hydrogen peroxide in body cavities. Hydrogen peroxide can be toxic to tissues as well as to bacteria—thus, after the initial "cleansing" application, hydrogen peroxide should not be used repeatedly on wounds because it may actually delay healing. For best results, do not apply an occlusive dressing immediately after using hydrogen peroxide; instead, allow the injured area to air dry first.[3]

• **Iodines (tincture of iodine, iodine solution, povidone-iodine).** Although all iodine products are irritating to damaged tissue, some are more so than others. Tincture of iodine is the most irritating, followed by iodine solution, and then povidone-iodine (Betadine). The least irritat-ing—povidone-iodine—is also the least effective of the three. To avoid intensifying the potential for skin irritation, you should not apply an occlusive dressing to the wound after applying iodine. Iodine stains the skin (and anything else it comes into contact with), so you must be careful when applying it.[3] Note that the IgE antibody mediated seafood allergy has never been attributed to iodine, but rather to specific proteins in fish and shellfish.[6] Therefore, a fish or shellfish allergy does not indicate a sensitivity or allergy to iodine.

Antibiotics

Antibiotics are substances that kill microorganisms and therefore treat as well as prevent infections. Antibiotics are biological by-products, usually made from cultures of the actual microorganisms they are intended to destroy. Bacitracin zinc, neomycin, and polymyxin B sulfate are examples of topical antibiotics.

Indications and Uses

Topical antibiotics can often be used instead of oral antibiotics for minor skin infections. Advantages to using a topical antibiotic in place of systemic therapy include fewer side effects, no risk of drug interactions, and less likelihood of drug resistance. Topical antibiotics are formulated as ointments, creams, powders, and aerosols. You should apply them only to small areas of the skin; using them on wider areas of broken skin can lead to systemic absorption of the active ingredients and a toxic reaction in susceptible individuals.

Individual antibiotics are specific to a range of species of bacteria; therefore, the antibiotic that treats *Streptococcus* bacteria may have no effect on *Staphylococcus* bacteria. Since it can be difficult to predict which types of bacteria might infect a wound, you should choose an antibiotic product that combines several active ingredients. Each additional antibiotic in the product extends the spectrum of bacteria that the product will control. If pain relief is a consideration along with the treatment of infection, choose combination products with names that incorporate the suffix *caine* or *amine*, which indicates the presence of a topical anesthetic.[8] (See chapter 6 for additional information.)

General Dose Protocols

A clean, bloodless cut may need no further treatment beyond simple soap and water if the skin around the wound is mostly intact and in normal position. A scraped knee or elbow, though, may require additional treatment to kill any microorganisms that may have entered the wound along with dirt and other debris. Although it is not harmful to apply both an antiseptic and an antibiotic, this is generally not necessary. Keeping a skin wound moist by wrapping it with a light dressing helps promote healing; however, not all wounds require the application of a topical antibiotic. If properly cleansed with soap and water, uncontaminated skin wounds rarely require a topical antibiotic.

When topical antibiotics are needed, you should use them only in small amounts and never for more than 1 week unless a physician recommends otherwise. Apply a small amount of ointment or cream—an amount approximately equal in size to the surface area on the tip of your finger—one to three times daily and cover the area with a sterile bandage. If the antibiotic is in powder form, apply a light dusting directly on the wound; if it is in aerosol form, spray a small amount on the wound.[8]

Distinguishing Features

Topical antibiotics that are available without a prescription generally contain one or more of the following substances as their primary active ingredients:

- **Bacitracin zinc (Baciguent).** Bacitracin zinc kills bacteria by blocking their ability to build cellular walls. It is mainly effective against *Staphylococcus* and other gram-positive bacteria, as well as some gram-negative bacteria or fungi.* Bacitracin zinc is generally considered safe, although significant amounts absorbed systemically can cause nephrotoxicity; hypersensitivity is also a possibility.[8]

- **Neomycin (Myciguent).** Neomycin belongs to a class of antibiotics called *aminoglycosides,* which effectively kill bacteria by interfering with their ability to synthesize protein. Neomycin is effective against *Staphylococcus* and some gram-negative bacteria but not against fungi. Keep in mind, too, that neomycin can cause hypersensitivity reactions. When used in large amounts and absorbed systemically, neomycin can also cause nephrotoxicity and may damage hearing.[8]

- **Polymyxin B sulfate (approved for use in combination products only).** Polymyxin B sulfate is a useful companion to bacitracin and other antibiotics that are effective against gram-positive organisms. Polymyxin B sulfate is effective against gram-negative bacteria but not against *Staphylococcus* or fungi. This antibiotic can cause nephrotoxicity, but only in rare instances when applied topically in large amounts.[8]

- **Combination products.** Many different types of bacteria can infect a wound, and individual antibiotics are specific to individual bacteria; therefore, a proper course of treatment in most cases involves the use of a topical antibiotic that combines two or more different active ingredients. Topical combination products that are commonly used and are available without a prescription include Neosporin (contains bacitracin zinc, neomycin, and polymyxin B sulfate) and Polysporin (contains bacitracin zinc and polymyxin B sulfate). Generic versions of these brand-name products are also available over the counter.

Antifungals

Antifungals are another type of substance that can be used to treat infections, but only those infections caused specifically by fungal cells. These cells are plantlike microorganisms that lack chlorophyll (the green pigment) and must therefore derive their life energy from other living things rather than from the sun. In humans, fungal *molds* cause such conditions as athlete's foot, jock itch, and ringworm; fungal *yeasts* cause candidiasis and moniliasis. Tolnaftate, clotrimazole, and miconazole nitrate are examples of topical antifungals.

Indications and Uses

Topical antifungals are an appropriate choice only when you know that the infection and resulting skin eruptions are caused by fungal cells. In humans, these cells take the form of either molds or yeasts.

Fungal infections are typically itchy and red, and they may become painful if the skin cracks, allowing bacteria to enter and cause a secondary infection. In severe cases, the affected tissue may exhibit the

---

* The terms *gram-positive* and *gram-negative* are used to describe a bacterial organism's penchant for absorbing a dye called "Gram's stain" that colors the organism purple and renders it visible under a microscope. Organisms that absorb the dye and appear purple under magnification are gram-positive; gram-negative organisms are those that absorb little or none of the dye and appear faint pink under the microscope.

appearance and odor of decaying matter. In some fungal attacks, a secondary eruption appears elsewhere on the body (called a *dermatophytid reaction*). This secondary eruption is actually the by-product of an overreaction of the body's defense mechanisms in which white blood cells attack skin that is not infected.

It is sometimes difficult for laypeople to diagnose fungal infections because many nonfungal skin diseases can create similar itchy, red lesions. If in doubt about a particular condition, or if self-treatment with an over-the-counter antifungal agent does not quickly relieve the itch or pain, you should encourage the athlete to seek medical attention.

The following fungal infections are common among athletes: athlete's foot, jock itch, ringworm, and candidiasis. In the following sections, you'll learn more about these conditions, how to prevent them, and appropriate treatments.

Athlete's Foot

Athlete's foot (tinea pedis) usually originates in the toe webs—particularly between the fourth and fifth toes, which are the closest together. This condition is characterized by a red rash that is dry, itchy, and scaly. As the condition progresses, the toe webs may appear white and soggy. Cracks, blisters, and pimples may also erupt on the soles of the feet, making walking painful. Athlete's foot is more common in men than in women, especially in those between the ages of 15 and 40. It is easily acquired in locker rooms and other damp locations where many bare and dirty feet are likely to tread.

Prevention is the best approach to athlete's foot, because once this condition takes hold, it may be difficult to cure. To help your athletes avoid contracting athlete's foot, encourage them to wash their feet one or two times daily with mild soap and water and to keep their feet dry and cool by wearing light, absorbent socks and well-ventilated shoes. Tell your athletes to always change their socks after their feet have perspired, as is typical during athletic activity.

Treatment for athlete's foot consists of applying an antifungal agent to the affected area twice a day. In more severe cases, a physician may also prescribe a regimen of oral antifungals. Symptoms usually abate within a few days; however, fungal spores can remain hidden in skin cracks and nail beds, so although the condition appears to have cleared up, it may not actually be cured. Once the original infection has cleared, physicians often recommend regular and continued application of an antifungal product as a preventive measure.

Jock Itch

Jock itch (tinea cruris)—which attacks the upper, inner thighs and groin area of men, especially those between the ages of 18 and 40—is characterized by a red, scaly rash that is quite itchy. Often, the rash has a ring-shaped or sharp border. This condition usually originates in the crease between the inner thigh and scrotum; if untreated, it may spread around the groin, down the thigh, and across the scrotum and penis. Women may also experience a similar condition, simply called *feminine itching.* In either gender, keeping the groin (or vulva) area clean and avoiding under- and outerwear that is airtight or that chafes will help prevent jock itch from developing. Once this condition takes hold, however, your athletes need antifungal agents to treat it effectively.

Ringworm

Despite its name, ringworm is not associated with worms of any kind. Body ringworm (tinea corporis) is characterized by skin eruptions that are scaly, itchy, red, and ring shaped. You can successfully treat mild cases of body ringworm with over-the-counter antifungal agents, but more serious cases may require medical intervention and oral antifungals. The related conditions of scalp ringworm (tinea capitis) and nail ringworm (tinea unguium) are more difficult to self-treat because over-the-counter antifungal powders, sprays, and liquids penetrate poorly to hair roots and nail beds. Thus, these specific types of ringworm usually require medical intervention.

Candidiasis

Not all fungal diseases of the groin and feet are caused by molds; some are caused by yeasts. The most common offender is *Candida albicans,* which causes the infection known as *candidiasis.* Yeast infections thrive in moist, damp environments. On the feet, *C. albicans* may cause redness, peeling skin, and cracking between the toes. In the groin, yeast infections appear as bright red, weepy rashes with pimplelike bumps that are itchy. In men, the rash may spread to the scrotum and outside the rectum; in women, yeast infections cause external itching of the vulva and a characteristic vaginal discharge. Risk factors for the development of candidiasis include diabetes, pregnancy, obesity, immunodeficiency conditions such as AIDS, profuse sweating, and the use of certain drugs (especially oral corticosteroids and broad-spectrum oral antibiotics).

It is often difficult to distinguish between a fungal infection caused by a mold and one caused by yeast. However, this determination must be made because many of the drugs used to treat infections caused by molds are not effective against those caused by yeasts.

Drugs needed to cure yeast infections have been available OTC for nearly two decades. Up until 1990, they were available only by prescription. In various formulas, tioconazole, clotrimazole, and miconazole nitrate are readily available for treating yeast-induced skin eruptions (external use) and vaginal yeast infections (internal use).

The FDA was initially reluctant to grant OTC status to anticandidal drugs because of doubts about whether women could self-diagnose yeast infections, particularly those that infect the vagina. The prevailing thought was that since these infections in women can be easily mistaken for other itchy conditions—including the less common but more serious trichomoniasis—misdiagnosis would often result in treatment with the wrong drug. Trichomoniasis, which is caused by the protozoa *Trichomonas vaginalis,* does not respond to tioconazole, clotrimazole, or miconazole nitrate. It must be treated with metronidazole, which is a drug that is available only by prescription.

However, after careful study and input from the medical community, the FDA concluded that women can successfully diagnose yeast infections themselves—but only on second and subsequent outbreaks. Thus, before allowing tioconazole, clotrimazole, and miconazole nitrate to be sold without a prescription, the FDA required manufacturers to include the following disclaimer on their product labels: "If this is the *first* time you have had a vaginal or vulvar itch with discomfort, consult your doctor. If you have had a doctor's diagnosis of a vaginal yeast infection and have the same symptoms now, use [this product] as directed."

General Dose Protocols

Athlete's foot, jock itch, and ringworm are caused by similar molds. So although these conditions invade different parts of the body, they generally respond to the same drugs. Topical antifungals for these infections are typically formulated as ointments, powders, creams, liquids, or aerosol sprays. The soluble forms (liquids and sprays) appear to be the most effective because they dry quickly and leave the antifungal agent in close contact with the skin.[8]

Before applying a topical antifungal for the treatment of an infection caused by a mold, the athlete should wash the infected area with mild soap and water. Normally, two applications daily—one in the morning and one before bed—are sufficient for these medications.[8]

Unfortunately, infections caused by fungal cells may recur because over-the-counter topical drugs may not penetrate deep enough to reach cells deep in the skin or nail. The FDA does not advise long-term use of OTC topical antifungal agents, particularly on injured or broken skin; the body can absorb the active ingredients in these products systemically through breaks in the skin, which may cause toxicity in susceptible users. As a rule of thumb, if a fungal infection does not clear up after a reasonable amount of time (2 weeks for jock itch, 1 month for athlete's foot or ringworm), the athlete should switch to a product that contains a different active ingredient or consult a physician. Orally administered antifungal agents are available by prescription only, and an individual may need one of these if the condition does not respond to nonprescription drugs. In cases where bacteria have accumulated along with the fungal cells, the individual may also need oral antibiotics.

Antifungal agents for the treatment of vaginal yeast infections are inserted into the vagina once daily at bedtime. The user may apply a small amount of cream topically as needed throughout the day for relief of external itching.

Over-the-counter products formulated specifically for the treatment of vaginal yeast infections are available either as creams (for use with applicators) or vaginal suppositories. Most are designed to alleviate the symptoms (itching, redness, and so on) within 3 days and to clear up the infection in 7 days. But some more potent variations of the same products, which combine cream and suppositories, are available for treating the infection within 1 to 3 days. Finally, an oral tablet (fluconazole, 150 mg)—available by prescription only—treats vaginal yeast infections caused by *C. albicans* in a single dose.

Distinguishing Features

Topical antifungals act by inhibiting fungal cell growth. Some are more effective than others; a few may be used to treat skin infections caused by either fungal molds or yeasts. All the products described in this section are available without a prescription. The FDA considers them to be safe and effective for use by adults and children over the age of 2; however, children under 12 should not use these products without parental supervision.

• **Clotrimazole (Lotrimin).** Until 1989, products containing clotrimazole were available only by prescription. Today, you can purchase this drug over the counter. Clotrimazole is effective against *C. albicans* as well as the fungal molds that cause athlete's foot, jock itch, and ringworm. The recommended dosage is a 1% concentration in a lotion or cream administered twice daily. Symptoms of jock itch and ringworm should disappear in 2 weeks, and symptoms of athlete's foot in a month.[8]

• **Miconazole nitrate (Micatin).** This broad-spectrum antifungal agent provides fast relief. It is highly effective against the fungal molds responsible for athlete's foot, jock itch, and ringworm as well as the yeast infections caused by *C. albicans*. The itching and burning that characterize these infections usually subside within 3 days. The safe, recommended dosage is a 2% concentration in cream or another base, administered twice daily.[8]

• **Tolnaftate (Tinactin).** Tolnaftate is considered to be safe and effective for treatment of jock itch, athlete's foot, and ringworm, but it is not effective against bacteria or yeast infections caused by *C. albicans*. Tolnaftate is the only OTC drug to date that has been proven safe and effective for *preventing* athlete's foot. One study showed a 90% cure rate in patients with athlete's foot who used tolnaftate.[8] However, this drug is not approved for ongoing use to prevent jock itch, because the groin is a much more sensitive area than the foot. You should consider a 1% solution applied twice daily to be safe and effective for treatment of jock itch, ringworm, or athlete's foot. People with athlete's foot may use one or two applications daily to prevent a recurrence once the initial infection has cleared up.[8]

• **Antifungal medications for treatment of vaginal yeast infections.** Multiple nonprescription remedies (Gyne-Lotrimin, Mycelex, FemCare, Monistat, Vagistat-1) are available for the treatment of vaginal yeast infections. These products contain the same chemicals (in similar concentrations) as the most effective products for treating athlete's foot, jock itch, and ringworm. Most are formulated as a vaginal cream with an applicator or as a vaginal suppository. The FDA considers the products to be safe for use by women who have been previously diagnosed with a yeast infection and are able to recognize the symptoms of a second episode. The course of treatment is generally 7 days unless otherwise specified on the label. If there is no improvement within the first 3 days of treatment, or if symptoms recur within 2 months, the affected woman should consult a physician. Women should not use these products during pregnancy or in combination with tampons.[8]

Antiviral Medications

Because of the complex nature of viruses, only a limited number of options are available for treating viral skin infections. The medications commonly used for the treatment of viral infections in athletes interfere with the virus' ability to synthesize DNA.

Indications and Uses

Only two topical antiviral medications are available for use—penciclovir (Denavir) and acyclovir (Zovirax)—and both require a prescription. These medications can be used to shorten the duration of symptoms following an eruption of oral herpes simplex lesions (cold sores or fever blisters). Viral skin infections seen in athletes include chicken pox (varicella), herpes simplex virus, shingles (herpes zoster), molluscum contagiosum, and warts. All are potentially infectious and may be spread by direct contact. These types of lesions are of particular concern in wrestlers because of the frequent skin-to-skin contact and the risk for transmission among teammates. Therefore, any new skin lesion in a wrestler should be evaluated by a physician before the athlete is allowed to return to practice or matches.

General Dose Protocols

Penciclovir is applied every 2 hours throughout the day (roughly up to nine daily applications), while acyclovir is used four times per day. Both medications are most effective when started as early as possible. This usually coincides with the initial "tingling" sensation felt before the eruption of a cold sore. Each medication is used for 4 days.

Distinguishing Features

Penciclovir and acyclovir should not be used to treat genital herpes infections and are not effective against other viral skin diseases. Shingles (herpes zoster) should be treated early in the course with oral antiviral medications (see chapter 7) because topical medications are not effective.

Several medications (e.g., salicylic acid) and remedies (e.g., duct tape, cantharidin) are touted as being effective in the treatment of molluscum contagiosum and warts; however, these medications do not have a true antiviral action. Although the actual mechanism of action of some of the remedies is not known, the salicylates function to incite an inflammatory response at the site of the wart, which then likely stimulates the body's immune system to eliminate the virus.

Considerations Before Use

Generally, all the topical agents covered in this chapter—antiseptics, antibiotics, antifungals, and antivirals—are safe when used as directed. Some of the topical antibiotics can cause serious toxicity if the body absorbs them systemically. But this is unlikely to occur unless large areas of damaged skin are treated. In addition, some of the topical antiseptics—alcohols and iodines, in particular—can be very irritating to damaged skin.

Systemic reactions to these medications are extremely rare. Athletes who are allergic to a given product may simply break out in a localized rash that may or may not itch.

Antifungals for treating vaginal infections are relatively safe. Rare side effects may include a worsening of the symptoms they were designed to alleviate: redness, vaginal itching, burning, and rash. Miconazole nitrate may also cause cramping, headache, and hives in susceptible individuals. Symptoms such as abdominal pain, fever, or a foul-smelling vaginal discharge are not side effects of antifungals. These symptoms may be indications of a condition more serious than a yeast infection. In such cases, tell your female athletes not to self-treat with OTC antifungal agents; they should seek medical attention instead.

With the exception of the antifungals specifically formulated for treatment of vaginal infections, all the products described in this chapter are intended for external use only. No one should ever use one of these products in the eye.

Common sense should prevail in deciding whether to bandage a wound. Occlusive dressings may increase the degree of systemic absorption of topically applied antibiotics and antiseptics. Dressings may, however, protect the wound and help keep bacteria from entering it.

All topical antiseptics, antibiotics, antifungals, and antivirals—including those used to treat vaginal yeast infections—may be used by athletes as needed, because none are currently banned by any governing body. However, WADA[7] and the NCAA[4] have different regulations regarding the use of certain medications, and these regulations are subject

---

TETANUS, a potentially deadly infection of the central nervous system, is caused by *Clostridium tetani* spores. None of the previously described antiseptics or antibiotics offers effective protection against this specific microorganism; immunization is the only preventative measure. The American Academy of Pediatrics recommends that children be immunized with the DTP (diphtheria, tetanus, pertussis) vaccine at 2 months, 4 months, 6 months, 15 months, and between 4 and 6 years of age. Adults who have been fully immunized should receive a tetanus booster shot approximately every 10 years.[1]

---

to change. For a complete list of banned substances, contact the appropriate governing body.

To use topical antibiotics and antifungals safely and effectively, you must employ common sense and follow package directions carefully. You should also make sure that your athletes do the same.

Guidelines for the Athletic Trainer

For most wounds, simple but thorough cleansing with a mild soap and cool water provides adequate protection against infection. Antibiotic creams or ointments are usually not necessary if you can immediately and properly cleanse the wound.

You can't get around the fact that tincture of iodine stings, but to minimize tissue irritation, you should avoid placing occlusive dressings over iodine-treated wounds.[3] Likewise, do not immediately apply a tight bandage to wounds treated with hydrogen peroxide—to be effective, this antiseptic must be open and able to release oxygen from the wound.

Neither topical antiseptics nor antibiotics provide protection against tetanus. For deep wounds and abrasions in athletes who have not had a tetanus shot within the last 10 years or who do not know their immunization status, experts recommend a tetanus booster.

All OTC topical antiseptics, antibiotics, and antifungals have an expiration date. Check the label, box, bottle, or tube and discard any product for which the expiration date has passed. Teach your athletes to do the same.

References and Resources

1. Centers for Disease Control and Prevention, National Immunization Program. *Diphtheria, tetanus and pertussis vaccines: What you need to know.* www.cdc.gov/vaccines/pubs/vis/downloads/vis-dtap.pdf. Accessed 11/15/06.

2. Cohen, P.R. 2005. Cutaneous community-acquired methicillin-resistant Staphylococcus aureus infection in participants of athletic activities. *South Med J* 98(6) (June):596-602.

3. Covington, T.R., R.R. Berardi, and L.L. Young, eds. 1993. *Handbook of nonprescription drugs.* 10th ed. Washington, D.C.: American Pharmaceutical Association.

4. National Collegiate Athletic Association. NCAA banned drug classes. www1.ncaa.org/membership/ed_outreach/health-safety/drug_testing/banned_drug_classes.pdf. Accessed 10/14/06.

5. Romano, R., D. Lu, and P. Holtom. 2006. Outbreak of community-acquired methicillin-resistant Staphylococcus aureus skin infections among a collegiate football team. *J Athl Train* 41(2) (Apr-Jun):141-145.

6. Sampson, H.A. 2003. Food allergy. *J Allergy Clin Immunol* 111(2 Suppl.) (February):S540-S547.

7. World Anti-Doping Agency. The world anti-doping code: The 2006 prohibited list. www.wada-ama.org/rtecontent/document/2006_LIST.pdf. Accessed 10/14/06.

8. Zimmerman, D.R. 1992. *Zimmerman's guide to nonprescription drugs.* 2nd ed. Detroit: Gale Research.

CHAPTER 9

Respiratory Medications

Respiratory infections are the most commonly encountered medical malady among athletes. These infections are typically caused by viruses and may result in a variety of symptoms that can affect athletic performance. Noninfectious respiratory conditions such as asthma and allergic rhinitis may also affect performance. If not properly controlled, asthma may not only affect athletic activity but can also be severe enough to require frequent hospitalizations.

Asthma—a Greek word that literally means *panting*—is a common, often serious disorder in which the smooth muscles that line the bronchial airways to the lungs tighten and go into spasms. This causes the airways to narrow and sometimes even become obstructed. When these spasms occur (a condition called *bronchospasm*), asthma sufferers experience tightness in the chest, wheezing, coughing, and shortness of breath.

Contrary to popular belief, asthma is not a problem of breathing in; it is a problem of breathing out. The underlying problem of asthma is chronic airway inflammation resulting in muscle spasm and edema in the bronchial tissues, thereby narrowing the small airways of the lungs. Thus, air becomes trapped in the lungs, making expiration difficult.

An estimated 16 million Americans have asthma; it is more common in children than in adults. Typically, the disorder is manifested in episodes that are set off by various environmental and infectious triggers. These triggers can include pollen, smoke, chemical fumes, and viral infections. Allergies—especially to pollen, grass, dust, mold, tobacco smoke, and animal dander—are the primary causes of asthmatic attacks. Less common triggers of the

KEY TERMS

allergic rhinitis

antitussive

asthma

bronchodilator

bronchospasm

decongestants

exercise-induced bronchospasm (EIB)

expectorant

bronchospasm associated with asthma include aspirin, exercise, and emotional stress.

Exercise-induced bronchospasm (EIB) is the term physicians generally use to describe asthmatic symptoms brought on by vigorous physical activity. Athletes may have asthma and EIB, or they may only have EIB. Experts estimate that 3 to 11% of athletes experience EIB.[3] For winter sports such as ice hockey, cross-country skiing, and ice skating, researchers have found incidence rates of EIB ranging from 14 to 50%.[8] In people with true EIB, exercise itself is one of the most common precipitants of asthmatic attacks. In people with any type of asthma, the prevalence of exercise-induced symptoms ranges from 40 to 90%.[2] EIB is usually short lived, in contrast to asthma caused by other precipitants. For some athletes, medications may be necessary; others can minimize the problem simply by avoiding exercising in cold, dry weather or by performing an adequate warm-up.[8] The underlying cause of EIB is not completely understood, but this condition can be well managed with asthma medications.

Asthma—whether induced by exercise or other triggers—is a potentially serious condition that should not be self-diagnosed. Thus, you must recommend medical evaluation to ensure proper treatment. A variety of OTC asthma medications are currently available (e.g., Bronkaid, VasoPro, Primatene Mist). However, any athlete with asthma symptoms should never use these OTC antiasthma medications and must be evaluated by a physician before being allowed to compete in practices or games.

Rhinitis is defined as inflammation of the membranes of the nasal passages. However, allergic rhinitis involves inflammation of the mucous membranes of the nose as well as the eyes, ears, sinuses, and pharynx. Symptoms include any of the following: sneezing, nasal congestion, nasal itching, and rhinorrhea (runny nose). The inflammatory response is always triggered by the immune system's response to a foreign protein or allergen. When the mucous membranes interact with an allergen, an inflammatory response is triggered that includes the immediate release of histamine and other inflammatory mediators, such as prostaglandins and leukotrienes.

Upper-respiratory infections (URIs)—also known as the *common cold*—are caused by several different types of viruses that directly invade the mucosal linings of the upper-respiratory system. After an incubation period of several days, symptoms begin as the immune system releases inflammatory mediators to fight the infection. Symptoms can be similar to those seen in allergic rhinitis, but they are typically more severe and may also include fever. Since virus subtypes are constantly changing, the immune system rarely sees the same virus twice. This leads to the possibility of a person experiencing multiple URIs throughout the fall and winter.

Lower respiratory tract infections can be either bacterial or viral in origin. These infections represent a more serious illness than a simple URI because of the involvement of the lungs (pneumonia). Such infections often require antibiotic treatment, which was discussed in chapter 7.

Asthma Medications

The muscle spasms that cause a narrowing of air passages during asthmatic episodes rarely abate on their own accord. In most cases, the athlete will need a bronchodilator—a drug that relaxes the muscles and expands the airways—to relieve the attendant wheezing and shortness of breath. In more severe asthma exacerbations, oral corticosteroids may be needed to treat the underlying airway inflammation.

Bronchodilators are available in a variety of formulations and strengths. Albuterol is the mainstay of asthma treatment. It is a beta-2 agonist that causes relaxation of the bronchial smooth muscles. Beta-2 agonists are available in short-acting and long-acting forms. Long-acting beta-2 agonists require several hours to take effect. Thus, they are indicated for maintenance therapy and are contraindicated for acute asthma attacks.

Indications and Uses

Many prescription drugs provide some degree of relief for the wheezing, coughing, and shortness of breath that characterize asthmatic episodes. Table 9.1 shows the effectiveness of each medication in acute and chronic situations. Athletes with EIB or intermittent asthma symptoms can typically manage their condition with the use of an inhaled beta-2 agonist delivered through a metered-dose inhaler (MDI) on an as-needed basis. Individuals with more frequent asthma symptoms will need to use an inhaled corticosteroid on a daily basis. In more severe exacerbations of asthma, a nebulizer is used to aerosolize the medication so that it can be slowly inhaled over several minutes. Oral corticosteroids are used for acute exacerbations of symptoms. Long-acting beta-2 agonists and leukotriene receptor antagonists are used to augment inhaled corticosteroids. Oral forms of beta-2 agonists are also available, but these have much poorer efficacy than the inhaled medications and more frequent systemic side effects. Thus, the oral medications should not be used in athletes.

Physicians prescribe several classes of drugs for the treatment and prevention of bronchospasm. These include beta-2 agonists, cromolyn and nedocromil, leukotriene receptor antagonists, glucocorticoids, and theophylline.

Distinguishing Features

Several families of prescription-only drugs are used to treat asthma. The mechanism by which each brings about bronchodilation is described here.

- *Beta-2 agonists* cause bronchodilation secondary to relaxation of the smooth muscle of the bronchiole. Beta-2 agonists are divided into short-

Table 9.1   Appropriate Uses for Various Bronchodilators

	Acute asthmatic attack	Maintenance therapy	Exercise-induced asthma
Short-acting beta-2 agonists	+	–	+
Long-acting beta-2 agonists	–	+	+
Cromolyn, nedocromil	–	+	+
Leukotriene antagonists	–	+	+
Oral glucocorticoids	+	+	–
Inhaled glucocorticoids	–	+	+
Theophylline	±	+	–

Key:
+ = indicated
– = not indicated
± = questionable effectiveness

acting (albuterol) and long-acting medications (formoterol fumarate [Foradil], salmeterol [Serevent]). This difference is important because short-acting medications take effect in a matter of minutes and have a duration of action of approximately 4 to 6 hours. The long-acting beta-2 agonists take several hours to have an effect and may last as long as 12 hours. Thus, long-acting beta-2 agonists must not be used for acute asthma attacks. The long-acting medications are used for managing mild symptoms over long periods of time, and they can also be used to treat EIB when activity may last for several hours. Use of the short-acting beta-2 agonists often brings side effects consisting of increased heart rate, nausea, headache, and jitteriness. Recently, a medication containing just the left (or "L") isomer form of albuterol was developed and is now marketed under the name levalbuterol (Xopenex). Use of Xopenex results in a longer duration of action (up to 8 hours) and a decrease in the frequency of the unpleasant side effects seen with albuterol.

- *Cromolyn and nedocromil* prevent mast cell degranulation, thereby inhibiting the release of inflammatory mediators and the reactive process that leads to bronchoconstriction. Although these medications are very safe, they are not as effective as the inhaled corticosteroids. They are also limited in that they must be administered three or four times per day to be effective. Though the mechanism of action is not understood, these medications are also effective in the treatment of EIB.

- *Corticosteroids* cause complex inhibition of the inflammatory process. Since asthma is primarily an inflammatory condition, corticosteroids are commonly used for long-term asthma management as well as the treatment of acute exacerbations of asthma symptoms. A full discussion of the corticosteroids is presented in chapter 4.

- *Leukotriene modifiers* block the inflammatory effects of the leukotrienes. Montelukast (Singulair) and zafirlukast (Accolate) are oral medications that act as leukotriene receptor antagonists.

- The bronchodilatory mechanism for *theophylline* is unclear. Researchers have proposed that theophylline has an effect on adenosine receptors that causes relaxation of bronchial smooth muscles. Some have suggested that the drug also has an anti-inflammatory action. Because of its significant side effects and risk of toxicity—along with the emergence of inhaled corticosteroids and leukotriene receptor antagonists—theophylline's role in asthma management has been greatly reduced.

- The *anticholinergic medications* are short-acting inhaled medications that are sometimes useful for treating bronchospasm. They reduce airway constriction by blocking acetylcholine activation of smooth muscle cells. However, these medications are not as effective as the beta-2 agonists and are only rarely used in asthma treatment.

- *Omalizumab (Xolair)* is indicated for individuals with moderate to severe allergic asthma. This drug acts to block the release of human immunoglobulin E (IgE). The medication inhibits the binding of IgE on the surface of mast cells and basophils. IgE is present in large amounts when the immune system responds to an allergen. Thus, if IgE is unable to bind to mast cells and basophils, the release of inflammatory mediators from these cells will be blunted. Omalizumab is administered by subcutaneous injection.

Side Effects and Adverse Reactions

Coughing after inhalation is a common side effect associated with all forms of bronchodilators administered by inhalation, including beta-2 agonists, cromolyn and nedocromil, and glucocorticoids. For beta-2 agonists, additional side effects may include muscle tremor, jitteriness, irritability, and sinus tachycardia. Repeated use appears to result in pharmacological tolerance—with time, larger and more frequent doses may be required to achieve the same effects.[7] Glucocorticoids may also produce dysphonia (hoarseness) and oral thrush.[7]

Orally administered theophylline can cause nausea, vomiting, gastrointestinal upset, and sinus tachycardia. An overdose of theophylline can be extremely toxic, resulting in seizures and cardiac arrhythmias. Individuals on theophylline should have their medication level checked frequently by their physician.

Some controversy surrounds the effects of beta-2 agonists on athletic performance. For example, research has shown that clenbuterol, a beta-2 agonist approved for use in humans in some European countries, has strength- and muscle-building properties.[6] Although it is approved only for veterinary use in the United States, clenbuterol is sometimes abused by athletes and is banned by the NCAA[4] and WADA.[10]

Inhaled or nasal corticosteroids, mast cell inhibitors, and leukotriene receptor antagonists are not associated with any known negative effects on performance.

Although xanthines, such as theophylline, may increase the contractile force of skeletal muscle, researchers have not attributed any ergogenic effects specifically to theophylline. Theophylline possesses diuretic-like properties and may cause dehydration, which has been shown to adversely affect aerobic performance. Furthermore, researchers have found that chronic use of theophylline decreases endogenous erythropoietin concentrations—and correspondingly decreases hematocrit and red blood cell mass.[2] Although no one has studied the impact of this hematological effect on athletic performance, theories suggest a detrimental effect on exercise endurance.[2]

Banned Substance Status

As with many medications, the NCAA and WADA have different regulations regarding the use of beta-2 agonists. Until 1993, the NCAA placed no restrictions on their use; today, the NCAA allows only inhaled formulations. Because the FDA classifies some bronchodilators as sympathomimetics, the athletes who take antiasthma drugs should make sure that they are not ingesting a banned substance. WADA is even more restrictive, permitting only certain inhaled beta-2 agonists (albuterol and terbutaline), and athletes may only use those after filing a Therapeutic Use Exemption. WADA requires that all athletes using inhaled beta-2 agonists have EIB proven by diagnostic testing. All oral bronchodilators (including orally administered albuterol and terbutaline) are banned by both the NCAA and WADA.

The NCAA and WADA also have different regulations regarding the use of corticosteroids (glucocorticoids). The NCAA places no restrictions on their use, but WADA bans intravenous, intramuscular, rectal, and oral use. WADA requires a Therapeutic Use Exemption for inhaled corticosteroids, but intranasal use is permitted.

Cromolyn and nedocromil are permitted by the NCAA and WADA.

The NCAA and WADA often have different regulations regarding the use of certain medications, and those regulations are subject to change. For a complete list of banned substances, contact the appropriate governing body.[4,10]

Allergic Rhinitis Medications

Since allergic rhinitis results from the release of histamine and inflammatory mediators, the mainstays of treatment have been antihistamines and steroidal nasal sprays, with leukotriene receptor antagonists playing an increasing role. A variety of preparations are available OTC and by prescription to treat both the nasal and ocular symptoms triggered by allergens. Oral and nasal decongestants are also used to control associated rhinorrhea.

Indications and Uses

Mild allergic symptoms can often be ignored. However, as nasal and eye irritation worsens, allergic rhinitis can make the affected person quite uncomfortable. The release of inflammatory mediators may even result in constitutional symptoms such as headache and fatigue. Although many people with allergies have multiple symptoms, some may have only eye or nasal involvement. Multiple prescription and OTC medications are available to treat allergic rhinitis (see table 9.2).

Oral antihistamines are commonly used for systemic therapy, but antihistamines are also available for use in the eyes and nasal passages. Leukotriene receptor antagonists have proven to be useful in the treatment of allergic rhinitis and have limited side effects. Nasal corticosteroids (see chapter 4) are also widely used to treat allergic rhinitis. Other nasal preparations include antihistamines (as mentioned) and mast cell inhibitors. If symptoms are only affecting one area, then topical use is preferable to oral because it avoids any systemic side effects.

Distinguishing Features

- *Oral antihistamines* are used as first-line treatment for the symptoms of allergic rhinitis. In an allergic reaction, histamine is released from mast cells, resulting in blood vessel dilation and inflammation. This leads to boggy, edematous nasal mucosa. First-generation antihistamines such as diphenhydramine are quite effective in treating allergic rhinitis; however, they have a short duration of action and can be sedating.

   The second-generation antihistamines are no more effective than the first generation, but they are much longer lasting (12-24 hours) and typically nonsedating. Topical nasal sprays are available OTC in the form of an antihistamine (Astelin) and a mast cell stabilizer (Nasalcrom). Antihistamines are generally not as effective as decongestants in treating URI symptoms, but the sedating effects can aid with sleep.

- *Nasal corticosteroids* are effective in decreasing the symptoms associated with allergic rhinitis. Multiple preparations are available by prescription (see chapter 4 for examples); however, none are currently available OTC. Since these medications are applied directly to the nasal mucosa, there are no systemic side effects. Their use can be associated with nasal irritation, dryness, and nosebleeds. They are not useful in treating the symptoms of URIs. Corticosteroid nasal sprays are discussed in greater detail in chapter 4.

Upper-Respiratory Infection Medications

Currently, no antiviral medications are available to directly fight the viruses that cause URIs. There-

fore, all medications are administered with the goal of relieving the common symptoms of URIs. All such medications are available OTC, including the following: systemic and topical decongestants, antipyretics for fever, analgesics for headache and sore throat, expectorants and antitussives for cough, and antihistamines for rhinorrhea and for helping with sleep.

Indications and Uses

Again, remember that all URI medications are used to provide symptom relief and will not directly affect the severity or duration of the infection. However, these medications may make the symptoms more tolerable. Topical decongestants are available to directly treat runny nose, while multiple oral medications are available to treat headache, fever, cough, and congestion. If a topical nasal decongestant can provide maximal simple control, then that is preferable to systemic use. Many OTC preparations combine several medications in order to treat the various symptoms that often occur with URIs.

The cough reflex results from irritation of the airway mucosa anywhere between the nose and the lungs. It may also result from nasal drainage into the posterior nasopharynx. Antitussives containing dextromethorphan or codeine are intended to suppress the cough reflex through a central action; however, their effectiveness is questionable.[5]

Distinguishing Features

- *Decongestants* are used to decrease congestion within the nasal airways. Congestion results from inflammation of the nasal mucosa. The decongestants are alpha-1 agonists; they act to bind to the alpha-1 receptors on blood vessels in the nasal mucosa and cause vasoconstriction. This leads to a decrease in blood flow to the mucosa and a drying of secretions.

   Decongestants are very useful in treating URI symptoms and can also be beneficial in treating allergic rhinitis. Several antihistamine and decongestant products are available OTC and by prescription (see table 9.2). Decongestants may cause side effects such as dry mouth and headaches. These effects can be avoided by using decongestants in the form of topical nasal sprays.

- Cough medicines such as *expectorants* are intended to thin mucus secretions and promote clearance by allowing a more productive cough; most *antitussives* suppress cough through a central action on the cough center of the medulla. The efficacy of either type of medication in management of acute symptoms is questionable.[5] Antihistamines

Table 9.2   OTC and Prescription Respiratory Medications

Medication	Rx or OTC	Common uses	Side effects
Decongestants			
Oral			
Phenylephrine (Sudafed PE)	OTC	URI, allergic rhinitis	Dry mouth, headache
Pseudoephedrine (Actifed, Afrin, Sudafed)	OTC	URI, allergic rhinitis	Dry mouth, headache
Nasal			
Oxymetazoline (Allerest, Afrin, Dristan, Chlorphed)	OTC	URI, allergic rhinitis	Tachyphylaxis
Phenylephrine (Neo-Synephrine)	OTC	URI, allergic rhinitis	Tachyphylaxis
Antihistamines			
First generation			
Diphenhydramine (Benadryl)	OTC	Allergic symptoms	Sedation
Chlorpheniramine (Chlor-Trimeton)	OTC	Allergic symptoms	Sedation
Brompheniramine (multiple OTC preparations)	OTC	Allergic symptoms	Sedation
Hydroxyzine (Atarax, Vistaril, Vistazine)	OTC	Allergic symptoms	Sedation
Second generation			
Cetirizine (Zyrtec)	Rx	Allergic symptoms	Drowsiness*
Fexofenadine (Allegra)	Rx	Allergic symptoms	Drowsiness*
Loratadine (Claritin)	OTC	Allergic symptoms	Drowsiness*
Desloratadine (Clarinex)	Rx	Allergic symptoms	Drowsiness*
Nasal sprays			
Azelastine (Astelin)	Rx	Allergic rhinitis	Bitter taste, nasal burning
Cromolyn sodium (Nasalcrom)	OTC	Allergic rhinitis	Headache, nasal irritation
Ipratropium bromide (Atrovent)	Rx	Allergic rhinitis	Headache, dry nose
Cough medicines			
Guaifenesin	OTC	URI	Nausea*
Codeine	Rx	URI	Sedation, nausea
Dextromethorphan	OTC	URI	Drowsiness*

*rare side effect

and decongestants are often more effective forms of symptom relief. Benzonatate (Tesalon) is a local-acting, oral antitussive that has a local anesthetic effect on the respiratory epithelium.

Considerations Before Use

Many factors need to be considered when an athlete is prescribed an asthma medication. First, the athlete must understand how and when to use the prescribed drug. Proper use of an inhaler device is critical to asthma management. In cases of EIB, timing of the dose is critical as well, because a beta-2 agonist must be taken 15 to 20 minutes before exercise.

For athletes with more severe asthma symptoms (nighttime cough, frequent exacerbations), an inhaled corticosteroid is often initiated. These medications are administered at least twice per day. Further treatment typically involves adding a long-acting beta-2 agonist and a leukotriene receptor antagonist. Compliance with a medication regimen is often difficult for athletes with asthma. An individual with well-managed asthma should not have any symptoms of the disease. Unfortunately, if the athlete has no symptoms, he or she will often question the need to continue taking the medication. To improve compliance and make taking the medications easier, products are available that combine an inhaled corticosteroid with a long-acting beta-2 agonist.

Allergy medications must be used as prescribed, but they are often only needed during a particular part of the year if the symptoms are from seasonal allergies. OTC allergy and cold medicines should be used as directed on the package. Overuse of topical nasal decongestants can lead to tachyphylaxis, a condition that results in worsening rhinorrhea with medication use.

All OTC decongestants are relatively short acting and need to be taken about every 6 hours to control symptoms. Topical nasal decongestants can be used by people who prefer to avoid the effects of oral decongestants, such as dry mouth. OTC antihistamines offer several choices. First-generation antihistamines, such as diphenhydramine (Benadryl), are typically short acting (about 6 hours) and often cause significant sedation. Codeine could also have the same sedating effect. Second-generation antihistamines, such as loratadine (Claritin), have a 24-hour duration and are nonsedating.

The use of OTC cold medications has no known negative effects on performance. The sport governing bodies currently have no prohibitions against the use of antihistamines, antitussives, or expectorants. The permitted use of decongestants is somewhat confusing. WADA[10] has no restrictions regarding the use of OTC decongestants. The NCAA[4] currently allows the use of phenylephrine and pseudoephedrine, but phenylpropanolamine and synephrine are both prohibited.

Guidelines for the Athletic Trainer

• Athletes who suffer from EIB and have been given inhalers for treatment of this condition should administer their medication approximately 15 minutes before exercising. Albuterol and other beta-2 agonists take effect immediately following administration; an individual may use these drugs on an as-needed basis. If an athlete has EIB that is not responding to treatment with an inhaled beta-2 agonist, the athlete should be evaluated for compliance with the schedule and proper use of the medication.

• As an athletic trainer, you should be prepared for athletes to ask you multiple questions regarding OTC cold medications. Thus, you must be knowledgeable regarding which products help with particular symptoms. In addition, remind athletes that many OTC preparations are combination products that often contain decongestants, expectorants, and analgesics.

• Compliance with a medication regimen is always difficult for athletes with asthma. If the athlete has no symptoms, he or she will often question the need to continue taking the medication. You can play an important role in helping athletes stay compliant by frequently asking them about symptoms and medication use.

References and Resources

1. Sheik, J. Emedicine. Allergic rhinitis. www.emedicine.com/med/topic104.htm. Accessed 11/15/06.

2. Bakris, G.L., E.R. Sauler, J.L. Hussey, J.W. Fisher, A.O. Gaber, and R. Winsett. 1990. Effects of theophylline on erythropoietin production in normal subjects and in patients with erythrocytosis after

renal transplantation. *The New England Journal of Medicine* 323(2):86-90.

3. McFadden, E.R. Jr., and I.A. Gilbert. 1994. Exercise-induced asthma. *The New England Journal of Medicine* 330(19):1362-1367.

4. National Collegiate Athletic Association. NCAA banned drug classes. www1.ncaa.org/membership/ed_outreach/health-safety/drug_testing/banned_drug_classes.pdf. Accessed 10/14/06.

5. Schroeder, K., and T. Fahey. 2002. Systematic review of randomised controlled trials of over the counter cough medicines for acute cough in adults. *BMJ* 324(7333) (February):329-331.

6. Spann, C., and M.E. Winter. 1995. Effect of clenbuterol on athletic performance. *The Annals of Pharmacotherapy* 29:75-76.

7. Sterling, L.P. 1995. Beta adrenergic agonists. *AACN Clinical Issues in Critical Care Nursing* 6(2):271-278.

8. Storms, W.W. 2005. Asthma associated with exercise. *Immunology and Allergy Clinics of North America* 25(1) (February):31-43.

9. Meneghetti, A. Emedicine. Upper respiratory infection. www.emedicine.com/med/topic2339.htm. Accessed 11/15/06.

10. World Anti-Doping Agency. The world anti-doping code: The 2006 prohibited list. www.wada-ama.org/rtecontent/document/2006_LIST.pdf. Accessed 10/14/06.

CHAPTER 10

Gastrointestinal Medications

Gastrointestinal (GI) diseases are common in both the general public and athletes. Unfortunately, a common symptom such as abdominal pain may result from a number of diseases, many of which can be quite serious. Thus, you must always ask about additional symptoms, including fever, loss of appetite, pain with urination, diarrhea, or blood in stools. If additional symptoms are present, the athlete should be evaluated by a physician.

• **Peptic ulcer disease (PUD)** is a chronic inflammatory erosion of the GI tract mucosa, typically occurring in the stomach or duodenum. Although the cause is multifactorial, one factor in this disease is increased amounts of stomach acid, which exacerbates abdominal pain.

• **Gastroesophageal reflux disease (GERD)** results from backward movement of gastric secretions from the stomach into the esophagus. The exact cause of GERD is unknown, but it likely results from a combination of increased production of stomach acid, poor muscle tone at the lower esophageal sphincter (the valve that allows transit from the esophagus to the stomach), and delayed emptying of the stomach. The most common symptoms of GERD are heartburn, regurgitation, and nausea.

• If the colon is unable to sufficiently absorb liquids from the stool, **diarrhea** will occur. This may be caused by a variety of factors. Viral infections are the most common cause of diarrhea, but it may also result from bacterial infections, food allergies, laxative use, and the ingestion of certain foods. In addition to loose or watery stools, diarrhea may also be accompanied by cramping abdominal pain, bloating, nausea, or an urgent need to defecate.

KEY TERMS

antiemetics

antiperistaltic agents

bulk-forming laxatives

gastroesophageal reflux disease (GERD)

H2 receptor antagonists

osmotic laxatives

peptic ulcer disease (PUD)

proton pump inhibitors

• **Intestinal gas** can often be uncomfortable and embarrassing, resulting in belching, abdominal distension, abdominal pain, and flatulence. Although intestinal gas is caused by the normal digestion of certain foods, excessive flatulence can indicate the presence of irritable bowel syndrome, lactose intolerance, Crohn's disease, or other disorders.

• **Constipation** is strictly defined as the passage of fewer than three stools per week.[5] However, the occurrence of any hard or difficult-to-pass stools is typically considered constipation. The most common causes of constipation include dehydration and insufficient intake of dietary fiber. Medical conditions such as hypothyroidism and irritable bowel syndrome can also cause constipation.

- **Nausea and vomiting** are among the most uncomfortable of all symptoms associated with gastrointestinal illnesses. However, vomiting is thought to be a protective reflex to rid the stomach and intestines of toxic substances. Viral gastrointestinal infections are the most common cause of vomiting, but a variety of other conditions may also result in vomiting. Gastritis, GERD, appendicitis, gallbladder disease, pancreatitis, and head injury may all stimulate the stomach to expel its contents.

Much like the respiratory medications discussed in chapter 9, gastrointestinal medications are typically used for symptom relief. Numerous medications are available OTC and by prescription to treat a variety of GI conditions. Almost all classes of these medications are available OTC and are heavily advertised in the media. Thus, anybody with GI symptoms is aware that relief for those symptoms is available at the local drug store. This may lead athletes to initiate treatment before asking for your advice or seeing a physician. Also, athletes may be embarrassed to discuss symptoms such as constipation or diarrhea.

Peptic Ulcer Disease and Gastroesophageal Reflux Disease

Symptomatic relief for peptic ulcer disease (PUD) and gastroesophageal reflux disease (GERD) is provided by lessening the acidity of the stomach, either through inhibiting acid production or neutralizing the acid that is already present. For PUD, symptoms may also be relieved by coating the area of mucosal irritation with a protective medicine. Five main types of medications are used to treat PUD and GERD symptoms; these medications are described here and summarized in table 10.1.

1. **H2 receptor antagonists** block the production of gastric acid. This is accomplished by inhibiting the release of histamine from parietal cells. Histamine is then unable to activate H2 receptors to increase acid production. The H2 receptor antagonists are widely available OTC; these medications are very effective and have limited side effects. They are often used when typical "heartburn" symptoms are not relieved by antacids.

Table 10.1 Medications for Treating Peptic Ulcer Disease and Gastroesophageal Reflux Disease

Medication	Common side effects
H2 receptor antagonists Cimetidine (Tagamet) Ranitidine (Zantac) Famotidine (Pepcid) Nizatidine (Axid)	Nausea, diarrhea
Proton pump inhibitors Omeprazole (Prilosec) Lansoprazole (Prevacid) Rabeprazole (Aciphex) Pantoprazole (Protonix) Esomeprazole (Nexium)	Nausea, diarrhea
Antacids Sodium bicarbonate (Alka-Seltzer) Aluminum hydroxide (Amphojel) Aluminum hydroxide and magnesium carbonate (Gaviscon) Aluminum hydroxide and magnesium hydroxide (Maalox) Magnesium hydroxide (Milk of Magnesia) Calcium carbonate and magnesium hydroxide (Rolaids) Calcium carbonate (Tums)	Chalky taste, mild constipation, diarrhea
Others Sucralfate (Carafate) Metoclopramide (Reglan)	Constipation Nausea, diarrhea, tremors*

*rare side effect

2. **Proton pump inhibitors (PPI)** also inhibit the production of gastric acid, but they do it directly by blocking the release of hydrogen ions from gastric parietal cells. These medications typically have a longer duration of action and are often more effective than H2 receptor antagonists at blocking acid production.[1]

3. **Antacids** buffer stomach acid and increase the pH within the stomach. Unlike the H2 receptor antagonists and the PPIs, antacids have no effect on acid production. They typically have a rapid onset of action but a short duration. Antacids provide short-term relief, but they are typically not as effective as the H2 receptor antagonists and PPIs.

4. **Sucralfate (Carafate)** forms a protective barrier over areas of damaged intestinal mucosa. In an acidic environment, sucralfate forms a sticky, viscous gel that preferentially binds to ulcerated tissue. It is available only by prescription and is used in the short-term treatment of duodenal ulcers.

5. **Prokinetics** enhance GI motility and the transit of material through the GI tract. In the treatment of GERD, prokinetics specifically act to increase motility of the upper GI tract. Thus, they allow the stomach to empty more quickly, lessening the time during which reflux may occur. Metoclopromide (Reglan) is currently the most frequently prescribed medication in this class. It has no effect on the large intestines.

Indications and Uses

Several OTC medications are available to treat the symptoms of both PUD and GERD. Although PUD and GERD are potentially serious conditions, they may begin with relatively mild symptoms, leading the athlete to try OTC remedies. In addition, mild and intermittent GI symptoms such as an upset stomach may respond well to OTC medications. Athletes with frequent, persistent, or worsening symptoms of PUD, GERD, heartburn, or upset stomach should be evaluated by a physician.

Mild abdominal symptoms will usually be relieved by antacids. However, H2 receptor antagonists are recommended if antacids do not provide complete relief, or if the symptoms are controlled for only a brief time. PPIs provide longer-lasting and often more complete relief of symptoms than the H2 receptor antagonists. For PUD or moderate to severe GERD, physicians will prescribe a PPI because these medications often decrease acid production to the point of allowing the gastric mucosa to heal.[2] Sucralfate is well tolerated but is used less than the PPIs in the treatment of PUD. A major drawback of sucralfate is that it must be taken four times per day.

Side Effects and Adverse Reactions

The OTC and prescription medications used for the treatment of GERD and PUD are relatively safe, with few side effects. The H2 blockers and PPIs may cause nausea and diarrhea, but these reactions are rare. The use of sucralfate may result in constipation, while patients taking bismuth compounds must be warned that these medications can cause the stool to turn very dark in color. There is also a small risk of salicylate toxicity if the athlete is using aspirin in addition to the bismuth compound. Antacids can result in a variety of side effects ranging from diarrhea to constipation. Chronic, long-term use of antacids may result in systemic acid–base imbalances.

Diarrhea Medications

Antidiarrhea medications may be used to prevent symptoms and allow normal daily activity—or in more severe cases, to prevent dehydration (see table 10.2). Antiperistaltic agents may relieve abdominal cramping along with diarrhea.

Table 10.2   Medications for Treating Diarrhea

Medication	Side effects
Antiperistaltic agents	
Diphenoxylate and atropine (Lomotil)	Dry mouth,* inhibition of sweating,* potential for worsening invasive bacterial infection
Loperamide (Imodium)	Potential for worsening invasive bacterial infection
Bismuths (Pepto-Bismol)	Discoloration of stools, constipation, potential for salicylate toxicity if taken with aspirin

*anticholinergic effects

• **Antiperistaltic agents** inhibit intestinal muscular contractions, slow GI transit, and allow for increased absorption of liquid from the GI tract. Loperamide is the most commonly used antiperistaltic agent and is available OTC. Although it is a member of the opioid family, loperamide has no effects on the central nervous system. Lomotil is the trade name of the prescription product that combines diphenoxylate and atropine. Diphenoxylate is an opioid with the same mechanism of action as loperamide. Atropine is an anticholinergic medication that also slows GI motility.

• **Bismuths** are used to treat PUD, GERD, and diarrhea. The most widely known bismuth compound is bismuth subsalicylate (Pepto-Bismol). The mechanism of action of these compounds is not known, but it is thought to be secondary to the antiprostaglandin effects of the salicylates.

Indications and Uses

Mild to moderate diarrhea secondary to viral gastroenteritis can be treated with antiperistaltic agents to control symptoms and diminish the total number of stools and total volume. However, any athlete with fever and diarrhea, or with bloody diarrhea, must be assumed to have a bacterial intestinal infection. In this case, the athlete should not be given an antiperistaltic. For bacterial infections, an antiperistaltic may potentially allow the infection to become more invasive, because the bacteria may cause medication to spend more time in the intestines.

Side Effects and Adverse Reactions

Drugs taken for diarrhea must be used with a great deal of caution. Lomotil, with its anticholinergic effects, can cause dizziness, dry mouth, and skin rash. Lomotil may also inhibit sweating, so it should not be used when heat illness is a concern. Another potential complication of the antiperistaltic medications is that they may worsen the effects of an invasive bacterial intestinal infection. In many cases, diarrhea acts to flush the intestines of the infectious or toxic agent. By inhibiting the diarrhea, the medication can give the bacteria more opportunity to do damage, making the infection worse. Thus, antiperistaltic medications should not be used in the presence of diarrhea combined with fever or blood in the stools.

Intestinal Gas Medications

Antigas medications are available to treat symptoms as well as to prevent gas accumulation if it is linked to the ingestion of certain foods.

• **Simethicone** works directly on gas bubbles in the GI tract. It works as a defoaming agent and reduces the surface tension of the bubbles of gas. This allows the bubbles to be broken down and released through belching or flatus.[6]

• **Alpha-galactosidase** (Beano) is an enzyme used to prevent intestinal gas. It acts to break down oligosaccharides (sugars found in beans, whole grains, peas, and lentils). If these sugars are not available, they cannot be metabolized by bacteria within the colon, and no gas is produced.[3]

Indications and Uses

Intestinal gas may result from overeating (swallowing air) or ingesting certain foods (fruits, vegetables, beans). Although the symptoms resolve over time, the buildup of gas can be very uncomfortable. Simethicone is very effective in relieving the symptoms once they develop. An alpha-galactosidase (Beano) can be used to prevent gas formation caused by certain foods.

Side Effects and Adverse Reactions

The medications used for intestinal gas are safe, and they cause rare and limited side effects.

Constipation Medications

Constipation can be treated with medications such as bulk-forming laxatives, hyperosmotic agents, and saline laxatives, which all act to cause fluid retention in the bowel (see table 10.3). Stimulant laxatives act to increase the propulsive activity of the colon and promote stool passage.

• **Bulk-forming laxatives** promote the transit of stool by distending the bowel, which in turn stimulates peristalsis (contraction of the bowels). *Stool softeners* are used to prevent constipation by being mixed into the stool as it is formed—once in the stool, these substances act to draw moisture into the fecal mass. Both bulk-forming laxatives and stool softeners are more effective if the individual taking them maintains adequate hydration.

• **Stimulant laxatives** increase intestinal peristalsis by stimulating local irritation of the intestinal smooth muscle or mucosa. These medications should always be used with caution. If the fecal mass is hard or impacted, severe abdominal cramping may result.

Table 10.3   Medications for Treating Constipation

Medication	Side effects
Bulk-forming laxatives	Intestinal gas, diarrhea
Stimulant laxatives	Abdominal cramping, intestinal gas, diarrhea
Saline laxatives	Intestinal gas, diarrhea

- **Saline laxatives** are intended for short-term treatment of constipation; they may result in electrolyte disturbances if used for longer periods. These medications are composed of soluble salts (magnesium sulfate, magnesium hydroxide) that act by drawing water into the small intestines. *Hyperosmotic agents* promote fluid retention in the colon, as well. However, osmotic agents such as lactulose are not absorbed by the bowel and can transit through the entire GI tract, drawing fluid into the bowel and causing few side effects.

Indications and Uses

Constipation also results in abdominal pain and discomfort and can be best prevented through adequate intake of liquids and fiber. However, when constipation does develop, a variety of medications are available for treatment. Most athletes will best tolerate a bulk-forming laxative. The athlete should increase his or her fluid intake in addition to taking the laxative. Hyperosmotic agents may cause gas and cramping. Stool softeners are used to prevent constipation from developing; they are often used before, or following, abdominal surgery. Stimulant laxatives can be effective if used in conjunction with a bulk-forming agent, but they may cause significant pain and cramping if used alone. Several of the laxatives are available in the form of an enema for rectal administration.

Side Effects and Adverse Reactions

Laxatives used to treat constipation can result in abdominal cramping, intestinal gas, and diarrhea. Cramping may be severe when stimulant laxatives are used without the addition of a hyperosmotic or bulk-forming laxative.

Antiemetics

The symptoms of nausea and vomiting (emesis) appear to be mediated through the central nervous system. Two main types of medications are available to help diminish such symptoms (see table 10.4). Medications used for nausea and vomiting are typically referred to as antiemetics.

- **Dopamine receptor antagonists** are the oldest and most widely used antiemetics. Although their effects are complicated, the principal mechanism of these medications is a direct effect on dopamine receptors in the brain. These drugs also have some anticholinergic and antihistamine effects; thus, they may cause dry mouth and sedation.

- **5-HT$_3$ receptor antagonists** were introduced in the early 1990s and are widely used for treating chemotherapy-induced nausea and vomiting. They apparently have both central and peripheral actions. These medications are rarely used for nausea and vomiting caused by gastrointestinal infections.

Table 10.4   Medications for Treating Nausea and Vomiting

Medication	Side effects
Dopamine receptor antagonists Prochlorperazine (Compazine) Promethazine (Phenergan)	Dry mouth, sedation
5-HT$_3$ receptor antagonists Ondansetron (Zofran) Dolasetron (Anzemet) Granisetron (Kytril)	Headache, constipation

Indications and Uses

Prescription antiemetic medications should only be used after an athlete has been evaluated by a physician, because vomiting may be secondary to serious illness. The antiemetics often cause sedation, so they may actually help the athlete get some sleep, as well. Rectal suppositories are often the most effective route of administration, especially if the vomiting does not allow the athlete to keep any liquids in his or her stomach.

Side Effects
and Adverse Reactions

Treating nausea and vomiting with medications should also be approached cautiously. Vomiting in the absence of diarrhea may be a sign of a serious gastrointestinal infection or other disease process. The antiemetics all have few side effects; however, the dopamine receptor agonists often cause drowsiness.

Considerations
Before Use

The majority of the medications discussed in this chapter are widely available. Also, because of a great deal of television and radio advertising, these medications are well known to most athletes. Therefore, athletes are likely to try one or more OTC medications to relieve their gastrointestinal symptoms before talking with you or a physician.

Gastrointestinal diseases can be difficult to properly diagnose, even for the most seasoned physicians and surgeons who have a variety of diagnostic tools at their disposal. Gastrointestinal symptoms can be a manifestation of anything from anxiety or depression to infectious diarrhea or appendicitis. You must assess the athlete's current symptoms and previous symptoms, as well as the athlete's current response to the medications he or she is taking. If the symptoms are persisting or worsening despite taking OTC medications, a physician must be consulted.

Other than the potential side effects and adverse reactions previously discussed, none of these medications has any known negative effects on athletic performance. In fact, because they are all primarily focused on symptom relief, the administration of any of the medications discussed should allow the athlete to perform at his or her standard level.

Currently, the NCAA[4] and WADA[7] permit the use of all the gastrointestinal medications discussed in this chapter. Regulations regarding medication often vary between the NCAA and WADA and are always subject to change. For a complete and updated list of banned substances, contact the appropriate governing body.

Guidelines
for the Athletic Trainer

- Given the embarrassing nature of complaints such as diarrhea, intestinal gas, and constipation, athletes may not come to you at first—or at all—for these complaints. However, for symptoms such as heartburn and abdominal pain, athletes are likely to seek your advice. Abdominal pain is a frequent complaint and is typically benign in nature. However, it may be the presenting symptom of a more serious underlying disease.

- Always determine the frequency and duration of any complaint regarding the gastrointestinal system. Sudden, acute abdominal pain should always be evaluated by a physician. Although viral gastroenteritis may cause such symptoms, appendicitis could also be the cause. Young women with acute abdominal pain should be immediately evaluated by a physician for appendicitis, ovarian cyst, pelvic inflammatory disease, or tubal pregnancy.

- In cases of mild to moderate abdominal pain, inquire about other symptoms, including weight loss, appetite, fever, bloody stools, and pain with urination. With female athletes, always ask about menstrual history and the presence of vaginal discharge. If any other symptoms are present, the athlete should see a physician rather than use OTC medication for symptom relief.

- If the athlete comes to you with symptoms that persist after already self-medicating for more than a week, you should direct him or her to see a physician (even if no additional symptoms are present).

References
and Resources

1. Bardhan, K.D., S. Muller-Lissner, M.A. Bigard, G. Bianchi Porro, J. Ponce, J. Hosie, M. Scott, D.G. Weir, K.R. Gillon, R.A. Peacock, and C. Fulton. 1999. Symptomatic gastro-oesophageal reflux disease: Double blind controlled study of intermittent treatment with omeprazole or ranitidine. The European Study Group. *BMJ* 318(7182) (February):502-507.

2. Bixquert, M. 2005. Maintenance therapy in gastro-oesophageal reflux disease. *Drugs* 65 (Suppl. 1):59-66.

3. Mangus, B.C., and M.G. Miller. 2005. *Pharmacology application in athletic training.* Philadelphia: FA Davis.

4. National Collegiate Athletic Association. NCAA banned drug classes. www1.ncaa.org/member-ship/ed_outreach/health-safety/drug_testing/banned_drug_classes.pdf. Accessed 10/14/06.

5. National Digestive Diseases Information Clear-inghouse. Constipation. www.digestive.niddk.nih.gov/ddiseases/pubs/constipation/index.htm. Accessed 3/3/07.

6. Olin, B., ed. 2001. *Drug facts and comparisons.* St. Louis: Facts and Comparisons.

7. World Anti-Doping Agency. The world anti-doping code: The 2006 prohibited list. www.wada-ama.org/rtecontent/document/2006_LIST.pdf. Accessed 10/14/06.

CHAPTER 11

Diabetes Medications

Diabetes mellitus is a disease in which the body cannot effectively regulate blood glucose levels. The defining characteristic of diabetes is hyperglycemia (high blood sugar levels). The diagnosis of diabetes can be made if a person has a fasting blood glucose level of >125 mg/dL on subsequent days.

Type 1 diabetes results from the destruction of insulin-producing beta cells in the pancreas by an autoimmune process. Insulin facilitates the entry of glucose into most cells for both energy production and storage. Type 1 diabetes is typically diagnosed in children, teenagers, and young adults.

Type 2 diabetes is usually associated with adults, and it is frequently seen as a complication of obesity. Because of the combination of increasing obesity rates and increasing recognition of the disease, type 2 diabetes is more frequently being diagnosed in teenagers and young adults. This disease can result from a variety of factors, including diminished insulin production, problems with glucose production in the liver, and insulin resistance in peripheral tissues. Since a more comprehensive overview of this common and complex disease is beyond the scope of this text, you may want to consult a medical textbook for a further discussion of diabetes mellitus.

Diabetic ketoacidosis (DKA) is the result of insulin deficiency. It may occur as the first sign of diabetes. It may also occur in a person with diabetes who is not properly managing the disease or who becomes ill with an infection. In the absence of insulin, tissues such as muscle, fat, and liver do not take up glucose; subsequently, blood glucose

KEY TERMS

diabetic ketoacidosis

glucagon

gluconeogenesis

hyperglycemia

hypoglycemia

insulin

type 1 diabetes mellitus

type 2 diabetes mellitus

levels rise. Counterregulatory hormones—such as glucagon, growth hormone, and catecholamines—cause an increase in fat breakdown and stimulate glucose production (gluconeogenesis). Beta-oxidation of these free fatty acids leads to increased formation of ketone bodies. Overall, the metabolic machinery of the body transitions from a normal "fed state" characterized by carbohydrate metabolism to a "fasting state" characterized by fat metabolism.[6]

The accumulation of ketone bodies causes the blood to become acidic. Signs and symptoms of DKA include hyperglycemia, excessive thirst, excessive urination, fatigue, blurred vision, "fruity" breath (secondary to exhaling acetone), nausea, and vomiting. Without proper treatment (insulin and intravenous fluid), DKA will result in death. Any athlete with signs and symptoms of DKA should be immediately seen by a physician.

How Exercise Affects Diabetes

Individuals with either type 1 or type 2 diabetes should be encouraged to exercise. In fact, for many patients, type 2 diabetes may be controlled with only diet and exercise, because exercise promotes weight loss and reduces body fat. Of course, type 1 diabetes always requires the use of insulin. Type 1 diabetes should never be considered a contraindication to athletic activity. Many college and professional athletes have been able to compete with proper management of type 1 diabetes.

Athletes with type 1 diabetes must carefully monitor their blood glucose levels and maintain a very strict diet and insulin regimen. At rest, only 10% of muscle metabolic requirements come from glucose, but with exercise, almost all the energy comes from glucose.[1] If insulin levels are low when exercise begins, the liver will begin to produce glucose, but the glucose will not be able to be transported into the muscle cells, resulting in hyperglycemia. Following exercise, muscle cells can take up glucose with the use of very little insulin; thus, individuals are at risk for hypoglycemia during this postexercise period.

The following guidelines are adapted from Dexter and Rahman[2] and should be followed by all athletes with type 1 diabetes:

- Estimate total caloric expenditure before exercise.
- Eat 1 to 3 hours before exercise.
- Inject insulin (away from exercising muscle) 1 hour before exercise.
- Ingest a snack if preexercise glucose is <100 mg/dL.
- Postpone exercise, check ketones, and increase insulin dose if glucose is >250 mg/dL.
- Consider checking blood glucose levels during prolonged exercise (longer than 60 minutes).
- Maintain hydration before, during, and after exercise.
- Have carbohydrate snacks available during and after exercise.
- Monitor glucose following exercise.

From W. Dexter and S. Rahman, 2005, Endocrine considerations. In *Sports medicine: Just the facts*, edited by F.G. O'Connor et al. (New York, NY: McGraw-Hill), 191. Adapted with permission of The McGraw-Hill Companies.

Types of Drugs

The primary goal in managing diabetes is attempting to maintain normal, or near normal, blood glucose levels. Although diet and exercise are important components of this management, medications often take a lead role. All individuals with type 1 diabetes require the use of insulin on a regular basis. Insulin is a powerful and potentially dangerous drug. Maintaining a normal blood glucose level always involves the risk of lowering the glucose level too much, particularly during exercise. To fine-tune blood sugar levels, many types of insulin have been developed. These types are divided into categories based on the time of onset and duration of action.

Type 2 diabetes may be managed with weight loss, diet, and exercise alone. However, if the disease process is more advanced, the person may require oral medication, and in rare cases, insulin. Currently, several classifications of oral antidiabetic agents are available (see table 11.1). The medications are classified primarily by the organ system where their mechanism of action occurs, though a few of the medications have multiple effects, and not all mechanisms of action are completely understood.

Indications and Uses

Once the diagnosis of either type 1 or type 2 diabetes has been made, the treating physician will decide on the best medication regimen to keep blood glucose levels within the normal range. Diabetes treatment involves a constant balancing act in the attempt to avoid both hypoglycemia and hyperglycemia. Insulin is always used in the treatment of type 1 diabetes.

In cases where type 2 diabetes is not controlled with weight loss, diet, and exercise, the individual must be placed on a hypoglycemic medication to lower blood glucose levels. In certain instances, people with type 2 diabetes may require insulin as their condition progresses. Oral antidiabetic medications may be used alone or in specific combinations, depending on a variety of factors.

Insulin

Insulin was not available for the treatment of diabetes until the 1920s. Before that, diabetes was a fatal condition. Insulin was initially extracted from the pancreases of cows, horses, and pigs. It is now synthesized through genetic engineering techniques, which have allowed the creation of a number of insulin forms with varying times of onset and durations of effect.

Table 11.1　Oral Hypoglycemic Medications

Medication	Mechanism	Side effects
Sulfonylureas *First generation* Acetohexamide (Dymelor) Chlorpropamide (Diabinese) Tolazamide (Tolinase) Tolbutamide (Orinase)	Stimulates release of insulin from the pancreas in acute treatment; mechanism of long-term function is unknown	Hypoglycemia, weight gain
Second generation Glyburide (Micronase) Glipizide (Glucotrol) Glimepiride (Amaryl) Gliclazide (Diamicron)	Same as first generation	
Meglitinides Repaglinide (Prandin) Nateglinide (Starlix)	Stimulates insulin secretion through a direct effect on the beta cells in the pancreas	Hypoglycemia, occasional weight gain
Biguanides Metformin (Glucophage)	Decreases gluconeogenesis; increases action of insulin in fat and muscle, which allows blood glucose levels to decrease	Diarrhea, abdominal discomfort, nausea, hypoglycemia
Thiazolidinediones Pioglitazone (Actos) Rosiglitazone (Avandia)	Increases glucose transport into muscle and fat cells	Hypoglycemia, occasional liver dysfunction
Alpha-glucosidase inhibitors Acarbose (Precose) Miglitol (Glyset)	Inhibits the breakdown of complex carbohydrate, targeting enzymes in the small intestine mucosa	Flatulence, hypoglycemia, diarrhea, abdominal pain

Rapid Acting

The available rapid-acting forms of insulin are insulin lispro (Humalog) and insulin aspart (Novolog). Both medications should be taken 0 to 15 minutes before a meal, and both mimic the insulin secretion process that occurs as part of the normal physiological response to food intake.[3] Along with their rapid onset, these medications have a very short duration of action (2 to 4 hours) and cannot be counted on to maintain blood sugar control for more than a short time.

Regular

Regular insulin (Humulin R) is a short-acting form with a duration of action of 5 to 10 hours. Because the time to onset is almost 1 hour, taking regular insulin before a meal may result in transient post-prandial (after-meal) hyperglycemia.

Intermediate Acting

Intermediate-acting forms of insulin—isophane insulin (NPH) and insulin zinc (Lente)—are commonly used, but individual responses may vary. This can result in fluctuations of absorption and thus glucose levels. Time to onset for these medications is 1 to 3 hours, with a peak level of action varying from 6 to 14 hours.

Long Acting

Insulin zinc extended (Ultralente) and insulin glargine (Lantus) are both long-acting forms of insulin. Ultralente has a very slow onset of action (4 to 6 hours) and cannot be used for the acute treatment of hyperglycemia. It is often used in combination with short-acting insulin to produce a basal level of insulin between meals. Lantus has no pronounced peak; therefore, it can be used to maintain a basal level of insulin throughout the day. Lantus is usually administered once daily at bedtime; Ultralente is administered two times per day.

Combination

A variety of prepackaged combination insulin products are available. These products typically consist of a mixture of short- and long-acting insulin in the same vial. These products require fewer daily injections and may help optimize blood sugar control and patient compliance.

Oral Antidiabetic Medications

As the prevalence of type 2 diabetes increases, the use of oral antidiabetic agents is becoming increasingly common. The sulfonylureas have been widely used for years, and a number of newer medications are also being used to control blood glucose levels.

Sulfonylureas

From a biochemical standpoint, the sulfonylureas stimulate the pancreas to release insulin. However, they have a far more complex effect on the treatment of patients with type 2 diabetes. Sulfonylureas cause an acute increase in the amount of insulin released from the pancreas, but with chronic administration, circulating insulin returns to pretreatment levels.[1] Despite this drop in insulin, the reduction of plasma glucose levels is maintained. The reason for this effect is unknown, but it may be that the reduction in plasma glucose levels allows circulating insulin to have a greater effect on target tissues. The sulfonylureas have traditionally been divided into two generations. There is no difference in the pharmacological activity, but the second-generation agents are considered more potent.

Alpha-Glucosidase Inhibitors

Alpha-glucosidase inhibitors have their effect on the digestive system. They specifically target enzymes of the small intestine mucosa, inhibiting the breakdown of complex carbohydrates. This action, when the drugs are administered with a meal that includes complex carbohydrate, may lower postprandial blood sugar levels by as much as 50 mg/dL.[4]

The biguanide class of medication consists only of metformin (Glucophage), which was first introduced in 1957. Metformin lowers blood glucose levels as much as 50 to 70 mg/dL. The medication is not an antihyperglycemic agent because it has no effect on the release of insulin from the pancreas. The exact mechanism of action is not completely understood but is thought to include a decrease in gluconeogenesis.[1] There also appears to be an increase in the action of insulin in muscle and fat, promoting the peripheral uptake and use of glucose.

The meglitinides are a newer class of medications that stimulate insulin secretion through a direct effect on the beta cells in the pancreas. Because of their quick onset of action and short duration of effect, the meglitinides can be taken with several meals throughout the course of the day.

Thiazolidinediones act to lower insulin resistance in peripheral tissues. They increase glucose transport into muscle and fat cells by enhancing the production of specific proteins that transport glucose across the cell membrane.[1] These medications also provide some regulation of the metabolism of free fatty acid in peripheral tissue. The thiazolidinediones are metabolized in the liver. Although their use does lower blood glucose levels, these medications also cause an increase in cholesterol levels. Prefilled syringes of glucagon are available for emergency use.

Routes of Administration

Although the mainstay of insulin delivery has always been subcutaneous injections, implanted insulin pumps have become more common. Usually implanted under the skin in the chest or abdomen, these small pumps deliver a small but constant amount of insulin throughout the day. They may also release preprogrammed boluses of insulin at certain times during the day to coincide with meals. Athletes with subcutaneous insulin pumps may have fewer problems with postexercise hypoglycemia because of the steady release of insulin. Athletes involved in contact sports must make sure that the pump is protected from potential damage.

The exact dosing regimen of insulin depends on the individual's weight, diet, activity level, and current response to treatment. Usually, several different types of insulin must be used throughout the day—in conjunction with a strict diet and frequent blood glucose monitoring—to ensure adequate control of the disease. Dosing of an oral antidiabetic agent is dependent on an individual's response to that specific medication.

Side Effects and Adverse Reactions

With insulin use, hypoglycemia is the most feared complication; it can also occur with some of the oral medications. Hypoglycemia can result from an excess of insulin but may also occur if glycogen stores are depleted through exercise or from skipping meals. Symptoms of hypoglycemia include drowsiness, weakness, confusion, dizziness, headache, trembling, sweating, and tachycardia. Any person with diabetes who has such symptoms should be assumed to have hypoglycemia. Ingesting 5 to 20 g of carbohydrate should restore blood glucose to a normal level and relieve symptoms. In severe cases, hypoglycemia can result in loss of consciousness.

If a person with diabetes is unresponsive, you must assume that the person has hypoglycemia, and you should give the person glucagon before activating the emergency response system. Glucagon emergency kits are available with a prefilled syringe of glucagon. If you take care of any athletes with insulin-dependent diabetes, you should stock at least one glucagon kit in your emergency supplies. Glucagon emergency kits must be prescribed by a physician.

Glucagon is a hormone produced by the alpha cells of the pancreas. Its role is to help the body maintain blood glucose levels. When released by the pancreas, or given by intramuscular injection, glucagon causes a release of glycogen from the liver and stimulates the liver to increase glucose production. Thus, if glucose levels are dangerously low, glucagon injection will quickly return them to a normal range.

Multiple injections of insulin at the same site may cause a buildup of fat tissue at injection sites. This is called *lipohypertrophy*. It gives the skin a lumpy or bumpy appearance. Rotating through different injection sites may prevent lipohypertrophy. The lesions can be surgically excised, if necessary.

Lipoatrophy results in a depression underlying the skin and is caused by the breakdown of fat tissue at the site of injections. The likely cause is an immune system reaction. The change in the underlying tissue may delay the absorption of insulin injected in that area.[4]

Insulin has been touted as having an anabolic effect on muscle, specifically if used in conjunction with human growth hormone. This interaction likely results from increased protein synthesis. Because of its potential use as a performance-enhancing drug, insulin is a banned substance that is tested for by WADA.[7] Athletes with diabetes who are dependent on insulin must file for a Therapeutic Use Exemption before competing at the international level. Currently, the NCAA has no restrictions on the use of insulin.[5] The lists of substances banned by the NCAA and WADA are subject to change. For a complete and updated list of banned substances, contact the appropriate governing body.[5,7]

For people using antidiabetics, the most common side effects of the sulfonylureas are hypoglycemia and weight gain. Because alpha-glucosidase inhibitors delay the digestion of carbohydrate, the use of these medications may lead to flatulence, diarrhea, and abdominal pain. Side effects of biguanides include diarrhea, abdominal discomfort, and nausea. Meglitinide use can result in hypoglycemia and may occasionally cause weight gain in some individuals. Thiazolidinediones are metabolized in the liver, so patients receiving them should have regular blood tests to assess liver function.

Guidelines for the Athletic Trainer

The athletic trainer must be aware of any athlete who has been diagnosed with diabetes. Since type 2 diabetes is more common in older and obese individuals, you will less frequently encounter athletes taking oral diabetic medications. Before the season, you should meet with the athlete who has diabetes (and with his or her parents if appropriate). This discussion should include a review of the athlete's medication regimen and the availability of snacks, glucose monitoring equipment, and glucagon at practices and games. You should also discuss procedures for contacting the athlete's physician in both nonurgent and urgent situations. You must also be well aware of the signs and symptoms of hypoglycemia, hyperglycemia, and diabetic ketoacidosis.

The athlete is ultimately responsible for his or her own health. However, as with any medical condition or injury in a young athlete, you should make sure that the athlete is complying with the established care plan. This should include regularly checking glucose levels, eating preexercise snacks, and taking insulin doses at the appropriate times. Periodically asking the athlete about blood sugar levels and diet can be helpful. Further inquiry may include sitting down with the athlete and reviewing his or her blood sugar levels over the previous 1 to 2 weeks.

If you have an athlete with diabetes, you should carry several carbohydrate snacks with you at all practices and games. (Examples of convenient snacks are dried fruit such as raisins, apricots, cherries; snack bars that contain at least 15 g of carbohydrate; juice boxes; and crackers.) Having your own blood glucometer may also be helpful, in case the athlete forgets his or hers. Also, although severe hypoglycemia is unusual in athletes, you should have a glucagon kit in your emergency supplies.

References and Resources

1. Davis, S.N., and D.K. Granner. 2001. Insulin, oral hypoglycemic agents, and the pharmacology of the endocrine pancreas. In J.G. Hardman and L.E. Limbird (Eds.), *Goodman and Gillman's the pharmacological basis of therapeutics.* New York: McGraw-Hill.

2. Dexter, W., and S. Rahman. 2005. Endocrine considerations. In F.G. O'Connor, R.E. Sallis, R.P. Wilder, and P. St. Pierre (Eds.), *Sports medicine: Just the facts.* New York: McGraw-Hill.

3. Holleman, F., H. Schmitt, R. Rottiers, A. Rees, S. Symanowski, and J.H. Anderson. 1997. Reduced frequency of severe hypoglycemia and coma in well-controlled IDDM patients treated with insulin lispro. The Benelux-UK Insulin Lispro Study Group. *Diabetes Care* 20(12) (December):1827-1832.

4. Mangus, B.C., and M.G. Miller. 2005. *Pharmacology application in athletic training.* Philadelphia: FA Davis.

5. National Collegiate Athletic Association. NCAA banned drug classes. www1.ncaa.org/membership/ed_outreach/health-safety/drug_testing/banned_drug_classes.pdf. Accessed 10/14/06.

6. Rucker, D.W. Diabetic ketoacidosis. www.emedicine.com/EMERG/topic135.htm. Accessed 12/3/06.

7. World Anti-Doping Agency. The world anti-doping code: The 2006 prohibited list. www.wada-ama.org/rtecontent/document/2006_LIST.pdf. Accessed 10/14/06.

CHAPTER 12

Circulatory Medications

For a person to maintain optimal athletic performance, the cardiovascular system must deliver oxygenated blood throughout the body, in addition to returning deoxygenated blood to the lungs (and metabolic wastes to the liver). Although athletes are typically well conditioned, they can experience a variety of cardiac and vascular problems. These problems may require medical management to allow an athlete to continue to participate in sports or recreational activities. In this chapter, we focus on medications that are used to treat hypertension and arrhythmias.

Antihypertensive medications are among the most widely prescribed pharmaceutical agents. People often assume that athletes and other physically active individuals are free of hypertension because of their high level of fitness. However, although physically active people are less likely than the general public to have high blood pressure, it is not unusual for even the most physically fit individual to require antihypertensive medication. Though not as frequently prescribed as the antihypertensive medications, several antiarrhythmic medications are available to treat individuals with abnormalities in the electrical conduction system of their hearts. Because of their mechanisms of action, two classes of medication are used for the treatment of arrhythmias and hypertension.

Antihypertensive Medications

Hypertension is typically defined as systolic blood pressure consistently greater than 140mm HG or

KEY TERMS

ACE inhibitor
alpha-blocker
antiarrhythmic medication
antihypertensive medication
beta-blocker
calcium channel blocker
diuretic

diastolic blood pressure greater than 90mm HG. Hypertension becomes more prevalent as people get older. As many as one-fourth of all people 30 to 60 years of age are hypertensive.[2] However, it is not an unusual diagnosis for young, active athletes—5 to 10% of people between the ages of 20 and 30 years have been diagnosed with hypertension.[5]

Indications and Uses

The goal of hypertension management—whether through lifestyle changes or medications—is to lower blood pressure to normal levels. Over time, untreated hypertension raises the risks for cardiovascular disease, renal disease, and stroke. Many patients initially diagnosed with hypertension are first managed with a trial of dietary changes and exercise to see if nonpharmacological intervention can control their blood pressure. Obviously, hypertensive athletes are already physically active, and many are already eating at least a moderately healthy diet.

Although several classes of medications are available to treat hypertension, all medications work under the same principles (see table 12.1). To decrease blood pressure within the cardiovascular system, one of three factors must be influenced:

1. **Blood volume.** Decreasing the total volume of fluid within the cardiovascular system will lead to a decrease in blood pressure. Conversely, in severely ill patients with low blood pressure (hypotension) resulting from infection or hemorrhage, intravenous fluids are used to raise the blood pressure.

2. **Peripheral vascular system.** If blood vessels in the peripheral vascular system can be relaxed, blood is allowed to flow more easily. If these peripheral vessels are less constricted, blood flow to the periphery will then be less inhibited. Medications used to produce this effect are often referred to as *after-load reducers.*

3. **Myocardial action.** Blood pressure can also be reduced by decreasing the heart rate or myocardial contractility. Any reduction in cardiac output will cause a concomitant reduction in peripheral vascular resistance.

When deciding which class of medication to use when treating an athlete's hypertension, the physician must consider certain factors. Some classes of antihypertensive medications may adversely affect athletic performance, either by directly decreasing heart rate and myocardial contractility (beta-blockers) or by increasing the risk for dehydration (diuretics). In addition, in collegiate and elite athletics, all forms of diuretics are banned, while beta-blockers are prohibited in specific sporting activities (see page 91 for further information).

Diuretics decrease plasma volume by increasing urinary output. They are divided into two groups: thiazide and loop diuretics. Both act on the kidneys' ability to reabsorb salt and water. Thiazide diuretics are considered less potent than loop diuretics and have fewer side effects. Potential problems with these medications include hypovolemia, hypotension, and hypokalemia (decreased plasma potassium level), which may result in muscle cramps and arrhythmias.

Loop diuretics are considered inappropriate for the treatment of hypertension in physically active patients. These medications can deplete intravascular volume and cause electrolyte disturbances, both of which may be exacerbated by intense exercise. Thiazide diuretics may be tolerable in patients with moderate levels of physical activity.

Angiotensin-converting enzyme (ACE) inhibitors block the conversion of angiotensin I to angiotensin II. Angiotensin II is a potent vasoconstrictor and promotes sodium retention.[2] The actions of ACE inhibitors allow for a decrease in total peripheral resistance and thus a drop in blood pressure. ACE inhibitors have no known effects that are significantly detrimental to athletic performance.

Because of their limited side effects, ACE inhibitors are considered first-line treatment in athletes with hypertension.[5] ACE inhibitors are contraindicated in pregnancy, so women of child-bearing age should use some form of contraception if they are on an ACE inhibitor. Angiotensin II receptor blockers are similar to the ACE inhibitors, but there is currently insufficient data regarding their effects on athletic performance.

Alpha-blockers block the alpha-1 receptors on arteriolar smooth muscle. This blockade causes dilation of the peripheral blood vessels and decreases systemic vascular resistance. The alpha-blockers have no known effects on training or sports performance.[1] However, because of a variety of side effects—including mild to moderate drowsiness, dry mouth, and impotence—these medications are infrequently used in athletes.

Beta-blockers significantly decrease heart rate and contractility of the myocardium. In addition, they can inhibit the breakdown of fats and glycogen, resulting in increased risk for hypoglycemia following exercise. Perhaps most important, athletes taking beta-blockers perceive greater exertion during exercise.[1] Beta-blockers may be beneficial to athletes involved in precision events such as archery, shooting, and billiards. Thus, these medications are banned in certain sports by both the NCAA[4] and WADA[6] (see page 91 for further information).

Calcium plays an important role in the contraction of skeletal and smooth muscle. *Calcium channel blockers* cause a reduction in calcium concentration in vascular smooth muscle cells, resulting in generalized vasodilation and subsequently decreasing systemic vascular resistance. Calcium channel blockers are generally well tolerated by physically active patients, having no major effects on energy metabolism during exercise.[1] These medications are sometimes used as first-line antihypertensive treatment in athletes.

Table 12.1   Partial List of Available Antihypertensive Medications

Medication	Mechanism	Side effects
Alpha-blockers Doxazosin (Cardura) Clonidine (Catapres) Terazosin (Hytrin) Prazosin (Minipress, Minizide)	Causes dilation of the peripheral blood vessels and decreases systemic vascular resistance	Drowsiness, dry mouth, impotence Note: These drugs are rarely used in athletes.
Beta-blockers Timolol (Blocadren, Timolide) Carvedilol (Coreg) Nadolol (Corgard, Corzide) Propranolol (Inderal, Inderide, Innopran) Metoprolol (Lopressor, Toprol) Labetalol (Normodyne, Trandate) Atenolol (Tenormin, Tenoretic)	Decreases heart rate and contractility of the myocardium	Hypotension, fatigue, exacerbation of asthma Note: These drugs are contraindicated for athletes and are banned in some sports.
Calcium channel blockers Nifedipine (Adalat, Procardia) Diltiazem (Cardizem, Dilacor, Tiazac) Verapamil (Calan, Covera, Isoptin, Verelan, Tarka) Amlodipine (Norvasc, Lotrel)	Reduces calcium concentration in vascular smooth muscle cells, causing vasodilation and subsequently decreasing systemic vascular resistance	Nausea, vomiting Note: These drugs are often used in athletes.
Angiotensin-converting enzyme (ACE) inhibitors Quinapril (Accupril) Ramipril (Altace) Captopril (Capoten, Capozide) Benazepril (Lotensin) Lisinopril (Prinivil, Prinzide, Zestril, Zestoretic) Enalapril (Vasotec, Vaseretic)	Blocks the conversion of angiotensin I to angiotensin II, which is a potent vasoconstrictor	Dry cough, potential interaction with NSAIDs Note: These drugs are often used as first-line treatment in athletes.
Angiotensin II receptor antagonists Candesartan (Atacand) Irbesartan (Avapro, Avalide) Losartan (Cozaar, Hyzaar)	Blocks the action of angiotensin II, a potent vasoconstrictor	Headache, nausea Note: The effects of these drugs in athletes are unknown, but the drugs are not contraindicated.
Diuretics Spironolactone (Aldactone, Aldactazide) Bumetanide (Bumex) Thiazides (Diuril, hydrochlorothiazide, HCTZ, Hydrodiuril, Oretic, Enduron) Triamterene (Dyrenium) Furosemide (Lasix)	Decreases plasma volume by increasing urinary output	Electrolyte abnormalities, orthostatic hypotension, dehydration Note: These drugs are contraindicated in athletes and banned in all sports.

Side Effects and Adverse Reactions

All of the antihypertensive medications have the potential to cause adverse effects. In fact, the avoidance of certain side effects often guides the choice of medication. The use of diuretics always runs the risk of fluid and electrolyte abnormalities. In addition, the loss of fluid volume can result in both dehydration and orthostatic hypotension (decreased blood pressure while standing). An annoying dry cough is the most frequent side effect seen with the use of the ACE inhibitors. Caution must also be used because adverse consequences can result from combining ACE inhibitors with NSAIDs. NSAIDs may blunt the antihypertensive effects of ACE inhibitors, and they may also affect kidney function. The risk of renal damage is increased if NSAIDs are combined with an ACE inhibitor and a diuretic.[2]

Beta-blockers have a variety of side effects—in addition to decreasing heart rate and cardiac output—that make them undesirable for use in athletes. Beta-blockers may exacerbate asthma symptoms and may also increase perceived levels of exertion during exercise. Calcium channel blockers have very few side effects and are well tolerated by athletes and physically active individuals. Because of unknown physiological differences, calcium channel blockers are often preferred over ACE inhibitors as first-line treatment in African Americans with hypertension. The alpha-blockers have no effect on exercise, but they may cause drowsiness, hypotension, and dry mouth, which makes them less desirable for use in athletes.

Antiarrhythmic Medications

Cardiac arrhythmias are a rare but significant problem that may afflict athletes. Different types of arrhythmias may result from various congenital or acquired conditions. All arrhythmias are caused by a disturbance in the discharge or conduction of electrical impulses throughout the cardiac tissue. If the heart is unable to maintain a natural rhythm, the cardiovascular system will not be able to maintain athletic activity. In some circumstances, the abnormal rhythm may deteriorate, and the heart may be unable to function, resulting in cardiac arrest.

If an athlete is diagnosed with an arrhythmia, the physician must first determine if the athlete can safely return to athletic activity. A variety of benign arrhythmias do not affect physical performance, such as premature atrial contractions and premature ventricular contractions. These may be felt as skipped heartbeats or may be found on a routine EKG. Other supraventricular and ventricular arrhythmias may put the athlete at risk for sudden cardiac death.

Indications and Uses

Although there may be some disagreement among medical specialists regarding who can compete in competitive athletics, general guidelines are available from the 36th Bethesda Conference.[3] As with the antihypertensive medications, when prescribing an antiarrhythmic medication, the physician must weigh the side effects that may have a detrimental impact on athletic performance while determining how to best control the patient's symptoms to allow activity.

In addition, many cardiac arrhythmias are managed without medication through the use of implantable pacemakers and defibrillators or through the ablation of abnormal electrical pathways in the cardiac tissue. Obviously, such non-pharmacological management is beyond the scope of this review.

Antiarrhythmic medications do not cure the underlying abnormality in cardiac conduction. These medications alter the underlying rhythm disturbance and allow the heart to return to full functional capacity. Because of their effects on important ions such as calcium and sodium, several of the antihypertensive medications are also used as antiarrhythmic agents. The following classification system categorizes the drugs by their basic electrophysiological properties (see table 12.2). However, you should note that even medications within the same class may have different pharmacological effects on the body.

Class I medications are sodium channel blockers. When conduction is inhibited in sodium channels, the excitability of cellular membranes is diminished. Less excitable cellular membranes will be less likely to conduct cardiac impulses through aberrant pathways. Medications that act as sodium channel blockers are divided into several subclasses. A further review of these subclasses is beyond the scope of this discussion.

Class II medications are beta-blockers, which were initially used to treat tachycardia but have been shown to be beneficial in the treatment of a variety of arrhythmias. The mechanism of action is unclear, but these medications may facilitate cell membrane stabilization by affecting sodium and potassium exchange. As we discussed for the antihypertensives, beta-blockers are poor choices for athletes because of undesirable effects on athletic performance (and because these drugs are banned in certain sports at both the NCAA and international level).

Class III medications block potassium transport across cell membranes in cardiac muscle. This affects the action potential of the membrane and disrupts spontaneous electrical conduction.

Class IV medications are calcium channel blockers that act to control heart rhythm by slowing calcium activity within the sinus and atrioventricular nodes. Only verapamil, diltiazem, and bepridil block calcium channels in cardiac tissue.

Side Effects and Adverse Reactions

In addition to the side effects associated with beta-blockers and calcium channel blockers (as

Table 12.2   Partial List of Available Antiarrhythmic Medications

Medication	Mechanism	Side effects
Class I Quinidine (Cardioquin, Quinora) Procainamide (Pronestyl, Procan SR, Promine) Disopyramide (Norpace) Flecainide (Tambocor) Propafenone (Rythmol) Tocainide (Tonocard) Mexiletine (Mexitil)	Sodium channel inhibition	Hypotension, potential for worsening arrhythmia
Class II See beta-blockers in table 12.1.		
Class III Amiodarone (Cordarone) Sotalol (Betapace) Dofetilide (Tikosyn)	Potassium channel inhibition	Nausea, vomiting, potential for worsening arrhythmia
Class IV Verapamil (Calan, Covera, Isoptin, Verelan, Tarka) Diltiazem (Cardizem, Dilacor, Tiazac)	Calcium channel inhibition	Nausea, vomiting, potential for worsening arrhythmia

previously described), class I and III antiarrhythmic medications carry an increased risk of actually worsening rhythm disturbances. For this reason, athletes beginning treatment for cardiac arrhythmias are closely monitored after medication has been initiated in order to ensure the medication is effective before returning to full activity.

Considerations Before Use

As previously discussed, the characteristics of particular antihypertensive agents may make them undesirable for use in athletes. Diuretics have too many undesirable side effects for consideration in the treatment of physically active individuals. Beta-blockers are rarely considered as therapy in athletes because of the inhibitory cardiac effects.

Thus, initial treatment of hypertension in athletes typically begins with either an ACE inhibitor or a calcium channel blocker. As discussed, ACE inhibitors are usually first-line therapy for the majority of athletes. However, NSAID use, the possibility of pregnancy, and the athlete's race (African American patients often respond better to calcium channel blockers than to ACE inhibitors) may result in the initial use of a calcium channel blocker.

The choice of antiarrhythmic medication is dependent on the rhythm disturbance being treated. A full discussion of choosing the proper medication is beyond the scope of this text, but you

should understand the potential side effects of the chosen medication.

Diuretics may be used to mask the presence of illegal substances by diluting the urine; thus, they are dubbed "masking agents" and are banned by both the NCAA[4] and WADA.[6] Although the side effects of beta-blockers make them a poor choice for treating hypertension or arrhythmias in competitive athletes, they offer a competitive advantage in sports that require a steadiness of hand. Thus, the NCAA[4] bans their use in riflery, while WADA[6] bans them in numerous sports, including gymnastics, billiards, archery, and shooting.

Regulations regarding medications may vary between the NCAA[4] and WADA[6] and are frequently subject to change. For a complete and updated list of banned substances, contact the appropriate governing body.

Guidelines for the Athletic Trainer

You must play several roles in the evaluation and management of hypertension in your athletes. First, the initial diagnosis is often made during preparticipation physical examinations. Thus, you may be asked by the team physician to measure blood pressure in athletes during such exams. You may also be asked to monitor blood pressure readings before and after medications have been started.

As an athletic trainer, you will have more frequent contact with athletes than most physicians will have; therefore, you are in a unique position to monitor and encourage compliance with any medication regimen that has been prescribed. You must also monitor the athlete's use of OTC and prescription NSAIDs. Blood pressure should be monitored daily in athletes with hypertension who are also taking an anti-inflammatory medicine.

Any athlete who has been diagnosed with an arrhythmia should be carefully monitored for the occurrence of any new symptoms. Any symptoms must be evaluated by the team physician or the athlete's cardiologist. You must also stay updated concerning the banned substance status of such medications.

References and Resources

1. Chick, T.W., A.K. Halperin, and E.M. Gacek. 1988. The effect of antihypertensive medications on exercise performance: A review. *Med Sci Sports Exerc* 20:447-454.

2. Gifford, R.W. Jr. 1997. Antihypertensive therapy: Angiotensin-converting enzyme inhibitors, angiotensin II receptor antagonists, and calcium antagonists. *Med Clin North Am* 81:1319-1333.

3. Maron, B.J., B.R. Chaitman, M.J. Ackerman, A.B. de Luna, D. Corrado, J.E. Crosson, B.J. Deal, D.J. Driscoll, N.A.M. Estes III, C.G.S. Araújo, D.H. Liang, M.J. Mitten, R.J. Myerburg, A. Pelliccia, P.D. Thompson, J.A. Towbin, and S.P. Van Camp. 2004. Working Groups of the American Heart Association Committee on Exercise, Cardiac Rehabilitation, and Prevention; Councils on Clinical Cardiology and Cardiovascular Disease in the Young. Recommendations for physical activity and recreational sports participation for young patients with genetic cardiovascular diseases. *Circulation* 109(22) (June):2807-2816.

4. National Collegiate Athletic Association. NCAA banned drug classes. www1.ncaa.org/membership/ed_outreach/health-safety/drug_testing/banned_drug_classes.pdf. Accessed 10/14/06.

5. Niedfeldt, M.W. 2002. Managing hypertension in athletes and physically active patients. *Am Fam Physician* 66(3) (August):445-452.

6. World Anti-Doping Agency. The world anti-doping code: The 2006 prohibited list. www.wada-ama.org/rtecontent/document/2006_LIST.pdf. Accessed 10/14/06.

CHAPTER 13

Neurological Medications

Medications for neurological conditions present a complicated topic for discussion. These medications often have complex mechanisms of action that are not completely understood. In addition, many patients taking these medications feel stigmatized and may not initially inform you about their medications. Therefore, inquiries regarding these medications should be made in private. Furthermore, some of these medications have a variety of indications for their use. For example, an athlete may be taking an antidepressant for bulimia or taking an antiepileptic drug for migraine headaches. Thus, you must specifically ask the athlete about the medical condition for which the drug is prescribed.

Many classifications of medications are used in the treatment of neurological disorders. Our discussion will focus on the common medications used to treat seizures (antiepileptic drugs), depression, and attention-deficit/hyperactivity disorder (ADHD). Because these drugs are widely prescribed, they are likely to be frequently encountered by athletic trainers. Additional neurological medications include those used to treat bipolar disease (mood stabilizers), schizophrenia (antipsychotics), and anxiety (anxiolytics). The neurological medications discussed in this chapter are only available by prescription. If you need further information regarding these medications, please refer to any current pharmacology reference.

Antiepileptic Medications

Antiepileptic drugs are used primarily, but not exclusively, for preventing the occurrence of sei-

KEY TERMS

absence seizure

attention-deficit/hyperactivity disorder

complex seizure

depression

epilepsy

generalized seizure

myoclonic seizure

partial seizure

seizure

simple seizure

tonic-clonic seizure

zures. Phenobarbital and phenytoin were widely used in the first half of the 20th century. The past two decades have seen an emergence of several new antiepileptic medications as pharmaceutical companies have strived to develop drugs that are more effective and less toxic.

Indications and Uses

A *seizure* is defined as a transient alteration of behavior caused by the disordered, synchronous, and rhythmic firing of populations of brain neurons.[4] Epilepsy is a disorder of brain function characterized by the periodic and unpredictable occurrence

93

of seizures.[4] Seizures are subdivided into partial and generalized. Partial seizures begin in one focal site of the brain, while generalized seizures arise from multiple parts of the brain. Partial seizures are further classified as either simple (where consciousness is preserved) or complex (which involves an impairment of consciousness).

Generalized seizures are divided into three types. Absence seizures involve an abrupt loss of consciousness associated with staring or cessation of ongoing activities, usually lasting less than 30 seconds.[4] Myoclonic seizures consist of brief shocklike contractions of muscles restricted to one or more extremities.[4] Tonic-clonic seizures involve a loss of consciousness and sustained contractions (tonic) of muscles throughout the body followed by periods of muscle contraction alternating with periods of relaxation (clonic).

In addition to seizure disorders, antiepileptic drugs have also been found to be effective in the treatment of varying diseases, such as migraines, bipolar disorder, ADHD, and chronic pain conditions. Don't assume that an athlete is taking a seizure medicine for a seizure disorder. See table 13.1 for a list of common medications used to treat seizures.

Phenobarbital (Luminal) was the first widely used antiseizure medication. This drug is inexpensive and very effective, and it has a relatively low toxicity. Phenobarbital appears to inhibit seizures through an action on GABA receptors in the brain. It is effective against generalized tonic-clonic seizures and partial seizures. However, this drug is no longer widely used because of sedative effects.

Phenytoin (Dilantin) was first synthesized in 1908, but it was not found to have an antiseizure effect until 1938.[4] This medication remains widely used today in the treatment of partial and tonic-clonic seizures. Phenytoin exerts its effect against sodium channels, slowing the rate of recovery after activation.

Carbamazepine (Tegretol, Carbatrol) is considered to be the primary drug used in the treatment of partial and tonic-clonic seizures. This drug appears to act by slowing the rate of recovery of voltage-activated sodium channels in the central nervous system. Carbamazepine is somewhat erratically absorbed after oral administration, so maintaining therapeutic drug levels can be problematic. Oxcarbazepine (Trileptal) is an analog of carbamazepine with a similar mechanism of action.

Ethosuximide (Zarontin) is the primary agent used for the treatment of absence seizures. This drug works by causing an effect on calcium currents in thalamic neurons.[4]

Valproic acid (Depakene, Depakote) has a mechanism of action on sodium channels that is similar

Table 13.1 Medications Used in the Treatment of Seizures

Medication	Mechanism	Side effects
Phenobarbital (Luminal)	GABA receptor inhibition	Sedation
Phenytoin (Dilantin)	Sodium channel inhibition	Problems with balance, behavioral changes, gingival hyperplasia, GI symptoms
Carbamazepine (Tegretol, Carbatrol)	Sodium channel inhibition	Drowsiness, vertigo, nausea, vomiting, aplastic anemia, mild to severe dermatitis
Oxcarbazepine (Trileptal)	Sodium channel inhibition	Drowsiness, vertigo, nausea, vomiting, aplastic anemia, mild to severe dermatitis
Ethosuximide (Zarontin)	Calcium channel inhibition	Nausea, vomiting, drowsiness
Valproic acid (Depakene, Depakote)	Sodium channel inhibition	Nausea, vomiting, potential for liver toxicity
Gabapentin (Neurontin)	GABA agonist (mode of action unknown)	Drowsiness, dizziness
Lamotrigine (Lamictal)	Sodium channel inhibition, other unknown actions	Rash, Stevens-Johnson syndrome
Topiramate (Topamax)	Sodium channel inhibition, other unknown actions	Fatigue, weight loss

to both phenytoin and carbamazepine. It may also have effects on calcium channels and GABA. Valproic acid is effective in the treatment of absence, myoclonic, partial, and tonic-clonic seizures.

Gabapentin (Neurontin) is a centrally active GABA agonist; however, its mechanism of action in preventing seizures is unknown.[4] This medication is often used in combination with other antiepileptic drugs in treating difficult-to-control seizures. Gabapentin is also used in treating migraines, chronic pain, and bipolar disorder.

Lamotrigine (Lamictal) has a mechanism of action that is similar to phenytoin and carbamazepine, but it likely has other actions because it has a broader spectrum of activity than those medications. Lamotrigine is used in the treatment of partial and secondarily generalized tonic-clonic seizures.[4] This medication is quite effective and is beginning to replace carbamazepine as a first-line agent.

Topiramate (Topamax) has a variety of effects on the central nervous system, including the reduction of sodium currents. This medication is indicated for use as a second agent in the treatment of partial seizures not responding to initial treatment.

Side Effects and Adverse Reactions

As newer antiepileptic drugs have been introduced, side effects and adverse reactions have diminished. However, finding the correct medication often involves attempting to gain control over seizure activity while limiting unwanted side effects. You need to be aware of the following potential side effects of the antiepileptic drugs:

- Toxic levels of phenytoin may cause problems with balance, behavioral changes, gingival hyperplasia, and gastrointestinal symptoms.

- Toxic effects of carbamazepine include drowsiness, vertigo, nausea, vomiting, aplastic anemia, and mild to severe dermatitis. Administration of the antibiotic erythromycin or the H2 blocker cimetidine can cause drug levels of carbamazepine to rise to toxic levels.

- Common side effects of ethosuximide include nausea, vomiting, and drowsiness.

- Almost 20% of patients taking valproic acid will experience transient gastrointestinal symptoms.[4] Valproic acid can also cause an elevation in liver enzymes. Fulminant liver failure has occurred, primarily in children under 2 years of age who are taking multiple antiepileptic drugs.

- Gabapentin is a very well tolerated medication, but it may cause drowsiness and dizziness.

- Lamotrigine has been associated with a sometimes fatal condition called *Stevens-Johnson syndrome*. Any patient who develops a rash when taking lamotrigine should contact his or her physician.

- Topiramate may cause fatigue and weight loss.

Antidepressant Medications

Antidepressants were first widely used in the treatment of major depression in the 1960s. As with the antiepileptic drugs, development of newer antidepressants has focused on limiting side effects while enhancing the mood-elevating effects of the medications.

Indications and Uses

Depression is characterized by clinically significant depression of mood and impairment of functioning. Symptoms of depression include persistent sad, anxious, or empty mood; feelings of hopelessness, pessimism, guilt, worthlessness, and helplessness; loss of interest or pleasure in hobbies and activities that were once enjoyed; fatigue and decreased energy; difficulty concentrating, remembering, and making decisions; insomnia, early-morning awakening, or oversleeping; and loss of appetite and weight loss or overeating and weight gain.

Tricyclic antidepressants (TCAs) were first developed in the 1940s. During the 1950s, several TCAs were used to see if they were effective in calming agitated patients with psychosis. Although they were ineffective in this capacity, it was found that they did have a remarkable effect on patients with depression.[1] The primary action of these medications is to block the uptake of both norepinephrine and serotonin in neurons. They also have other varied effects on neurotransmitters in the central nervous system. Many of the TCAs share a great number of similarities, but there are some differences in both actions and side effects. A detailed presentation of the differences among all of the TCAs is beyond the scope of this discussion.

Selective serotonin reuptake inhibitors (SSRIs) have largely replaced TCAs as first-line treatment for depression. The full mechanism of action of the SSRIs is not completely understood. SSRIs are designed to allow the available serotonin (a neurotransmitter) to be used more efficiently. A low level of utilization of serotonin is currently seen as one of the several neurochemical symptoms of depression. Though they are widely used, SSRIs are no more effective than the TCAs in treating depression; they are just thought to have fewer side effects.

Much like the antiepileptic drugs, antidepressants may be used for conditions other than depression. Antidepressants are often used for the treatment of obsessive-compulsive disorder, bulimia nervosa, ADHD, and social anxiety disorders. See table 13.2 for a list of medications used in the treatment of depression.

Side Effects and Adverse Reactions

Though effective, TCAs present a wide array of side effects, including dry mouth, heartburn, constipation, diarrhea, tachycardia, and arrhythmias. Other side effects include fatigue and weight gain. A major concern with prescribing TCAs has always been that an intentional overdose is often fatal. TCAs also interact with a number of other drugs, including phenytoin, aspirin, and alcohol. An athlete on a TCA should consult a pharmacist regarding the potential for adverse effects with any prescription or OTC medicine the athlete wants to take.

Although the SSRIs have fewer side effects than the TCAs, their use is not without problems. They present a high risk of nausea, vomiting, headache, and sexual dysfunction (mainly inhibited ejaculation or orgasm).

ADHD Medications

Given the large increase in the diagnoses of ADHD during the 1990s, ADHD medications have become widely used by high school students and are increasingly common in college students. The most widely prescribed ADHD medications are stimulants (derived from amphetamines). Methylphenidate (Ritalin) has been used in the treatment of ADHD since the 1960s.

Indications and Uses

ADHD is a common developmental and behavioral disorder affecting approximately 3 to 5% of children in the United States. It is characterized by poor concentration, distractibility, hyperactivity, and impulsiveness that are inappropriate for the child's age. Children and adults with ADHD are easily distracted by sights and sounds in their environment, cannot concentrate for long periods of time, are restless and impulsive, or have a tendency to daydream and be slow to complete tasks.

The stimulants used to treat ADHD (methylphenidates and dextroamphetamines) are structurally similar to amphetamines; however, they have

Table 13.2   Medications Used in the Treatment of Depression

Medication	Mechanism	Side effects
Tricyclic antidepressants Amitriptyline (Elavil) Clomipramine (Anafranil) Desipramine (Norpramin) Doxepin (Adapin) Imipramine (Tofranil) Lofepramine (Gamanil) Nortriptyline (Pamelor) Protriptyline (Vivactil) Trimipramine (Surmontil)	Blocks the uptake of both norepinephrine and serotonin in CNS neurons	Dry mouth, heartburn, constipation, diarrhea, tachycardia, arrhythmias, fatigue, weight loss
Selective serotonin reuptake inhibitors Citalopram (Celexa) Escitalopram oxalate (Lexapro) Fluoxetine (Prozac) Fluvoxamine maleate (Luvox) Paroxetine (Paxil) Sertraline (Zoloft)	Allows for available serotonin to be used more efficiently in the CNS (complete mechanism is not known)	Nausea, vomiting, headache, sexual dysfunction

more prominent effects on the central nervous system than on motor activities. The stimulants' exact mechanism of action in treating ADHD is unknown. It is thought that the stimulants have a direct effect on norepinephrine and dopamine levels within the brain.

The development of newer ADHD medications has largely focused on creating drugs that have a longer duration of action and maintain a steady level of drug in the bloodstream throughout the day. The first widely used stimulants offered only 3 to 4 hours of efficacy, so children needed to take multiple doses throughout the school day. See table 13.3 for a list of common medications used to treat ADHD.

Atomoxetine (Strattera) is the first nonstimulant drug approved for the treatment of ADHD. Because it is a nonstimulant, this drug does not fall under NCAA or WADA banned substance classifications. In addition, there appears to be no potential for abuse. Atomoxetine is classified as a norepinephrine reuptake inhibitor, and it is approved for use in children, adolescents, and adults. This drug can be taken just once daily.

Side Effects and Adverse Reactions

In addition to increasing the concentration and focusing abilities of people with ADHD, methylphenidates and dextroamphetamines exert their stimulant effects as well. Thus, major side effects include hypertension, impaired sleep, and decreased appetite. Suppression of appetite is the most important side effect to monitor in athletes. Amphetamines have been used for years as prescription appetite suppressants. You should consider regular weight checks for athletes taking a stimulant medication and consult a nutritionist if the athlete experiences undesired weight loss. The most common side effect of atomoxetine in adults is drowsiness, while children often experience upset stomach, nausea, and vomiting.

Considerations Before Use

The treating physician must consider many factors when prescribing medications for neurological conditions.

The diagnosis of a seizure disorder is typically obvious, and medication is required in order for the athlete to resume a normal life, let alone participate in athletics. There is often confusion regarding individuals with a seizure disorder and what activities they should be allowed to do. A seizure disorder does not automatically disqualify an athlete from participation. Guidelines from the American Academy of Pediatrics specify that an athlete with a well-controlled seizure disorder (no seizures over the past 6 months) may participate in a variety of conventional school-sponsored athletic events.[3] However, special consideration should be given to sports that may be considered high risk, such as high-apparatus gymnastics, high diving, and

Table 13.3   Medications Used in the Treatment of ADHD

Medication	Mechanism	Side effects
Stimulants *Amphetamines* Aderall Aderall XR *Dextroamphetamines* Dexedrine Dexedrine Spansules Dexostat *Methylphenidates* Ritalin Ritalin SR Ritalin LA Concerta Focalin Metadate ER Methylin ER Metadate CD	Direct effect on norepinephrine and dopamine in CNS, but exact mechanism of action is not known	Hypertension, impaired sleep, decreased appetite
Nonstimulants Atomoxetine (Strattera)	Norepinephrine reuptake inhibition	Adults: Drowsiness Children: Nausea, vomiting

skiing. In these circumstances, you should consult with a neurologist. Any athlete with a poorly controlled seizure disorder (seizures within the last 6 months) should be carefully considered for only a small variety of noncontact sports.

ADHD and depression are often more difficult to diagnose, because the self-reporting of symptoms by the individual is the primary basis for making the diagnosis. In some cases, the athlete may not believe that he or she needs to be taking the medication. Thus, patient compliance with the medication regimen may be an issue. If there is any question regarding the patient's compliance, two important factors must be considered in choosing a medication: side effects and dosing schedule. If an individual is questioning whether he or she needs the medicine, the occurrence of any side effect will provide a convenient excuse to discontinue its use. Also, a medication is more likely to be regularly used if it only needs to be taken once or twice per day.

The increasing use of stimulant medications for the treatment of ADHD is an area of uncertainty in the field of sports medicine. When given appropriate medication, young athletes with ADHD not only show benefits in the classroom but also display increased ability to concentrate on tasks during athletic practices, along with improvements in balance and coordination (perhaps secondary to improved concentration).[2] The ergogenic effects of these medications on this population are unknown. Athletes with ADHD should continue to take their medications as prescribed, regardless of athletic activity. The medication may be withheld during times of high heat and humidity in an effort to decrease the risk (albeit small) of heat illness.[3]

The majority of ADHD medications are amphetamine derivatives and, therefore, are banned by the NCAA[5] and WADA.[6] However, if athletes have a medical diagnosis of ADHD, they can file for a Therapeutic Use Exemption through WADA.[6] For this exemption to be granted, the athlete must be using a standard therapeutic dose on a daily basis; the athlete must also have been properly diagnosed by a licensed physician who regularly treats individuals with ADHD. The NCAA offers collegiate athletes a similar exception.[5] Currently, the NCAA and WADA have no restrictions on the use of antiepileptics or antidepressants.

Some regulations regarding stimulant medications may vary between the NCAA[5] and WADA,[6] and these regulations are frequently subject to change. For a complete and updated list of banned substances, contact the appropriate governing body.

Guidelines for the Athletic Trainer

Athletes may not want anyone to know that they are taking a medication for the treatment of a neurological condition, so you must assure them that their use of any prescription medication will remain confidential. Any athlete being medicated to treat ADHD who is competing at an NCAA or international level must file the appropriate paperwork to gain an exemption for stimulant use if drug tested.

If you are aware of any athlete taking antiepileptic drugs, you should be properly prepared if the athlete were to have a seizure. You should also formulate a plan of action with the athlete's personal physician or the team physician regarding what to do following a seizure.

Any athlete taking antidepressants should be closely monitored for symptoms of recurring depression.

References and Resources

1. Baldessarini, R.J. 2001. Drugs and the treatment of psychiatric disorders: Depression and anxiety disorder. In J.G. Hardman and L.E. Limbird (Eds.), *Goodman and Gillman's the pharmacological basis of therapeutics.* New York: McGraw-Hill.

2. Hickey, G., and P. Fricker. 1999. Attention deficit hyperactivity disorder, CNS stimulants and sport. *Sports Med* 27:11.

3. Koester, M.C. 2003. Making the preparticipation athletic evaluation more than just a "sports physical." Part 1: Bringing the history into play. *Contemporary Pediatrics* 9:85-103.

4. McNamara, J.O. 2001. Drugs effective in the treatment of the epilepsies. In J.G. Hardman and L.E. Limbird (Eds.), *Goodman and Gillman's the pharmacological basis of therapeutics.* New York: McGraw-Hill.

5. National Collegiate Athletic Association. NCAA banned drug classes. www1.ncaa.org/membership/ed_outreach/health-safety/drug_testing/banned_drug_classes.pdf. Accessed 10/14/06.

6. World Anti-Doping Agency. The world anti-doping code: The 2006 prohibited list. www.wada-ama.org/rtecontent/document/2006_LIST.pdf. Accessed 10/14/06.

GLOSSARY

absence seizure—An abrupt loss of consciousness associated with staring or cessation of ongoing activities, usually lasting less than 30 seconds.

absorption—The process that allows a drug to enter the body.

ACE inhibitor—Antihypertensive medication that blocks the conversion of angiotensin I to angiotensin II. Angiotensin II is a potent vasoconstrictor and promotes sodium retention.

add-on interaction—Occurs when an individual takes two drugs of the same type (e.g., two stimulants or two depressants) at the same time, creating a total primary effect that is much stronger than what is expected from either drug alone.

adverse drug reaction (ADR)—Any drug effect that is undesirable. May be classified as either local or systemic.

allergic rhinitis—Inflammation of the mucous membranes of the nose—as well as the eyes, ears, sinuses, and pharynx—triggered by exposure to an allergen.

alpha-blocker—Antihypertensive medication that blocks the alpha-1 receptors on arteriolar smooth muscle. This blockade causes dilation of the peripheral blood vessels and decreases systemic vascular resistance.

anabolic steroids—Derivatives of the male reproductive hormone testosterone, sometimes used by athletes as a performance-enhancing drug to increase muscle size and strength.

analgesic—A medication intended to reduce the sensation of pain.

antiarrhythmic medication—A medication used to control the occurrence of abnormal conduction in cardiac muscle cells.

antiemetics—Drugs used to inhibit the vomiting reflex.

antihypertensive medication—A medication used to lower systemic blood pressure.

anti-inflammatory—A medication that inhibits the body's inflammatory response.

antiperistaltic agents—Substances that inhibit intestinal muscular contractions, slow GI transit,

and allow for increased absorption of liquid from the GI tract.

antiplatelet—A drug that interferes with the blood's ability to clot by preventing the production of thromboxane, a powerful stimulator of blood platelet activation.

antipyretic—A medication used to reduce fever.

antiseptics—Externally applied agents that stop the growth of microorganisms. They are usually made from disinfectant chemicals that destroy bacteria on contact before the microorganisms have a chance to cause infection.

antitussive—A drug intended to suppress the cough reflex.

asthma—A Greek word that literally means *panting*. Asthma is a common, often serious disorder in which the smooth muscles that line the bronchial airways to the lungs tighten and go into spasms, thereby causing the airways to narrow and sometimes even become obstructed.

athlete's foot—A fungal infection of the feet (tinea pedis) that usually manifests with cracking and itching of the skin between the toes.

attention-deficit/hyperactivity disorder—A disorder characterized by poor concentration, distractibility, hyperactivity, and impulsiveness that are inappropriate for the child's age.

beta-blocker—Antihypertensive medication that significantly decreases heart rate and contractility of the myocardium.

bioavailability—The amount of a drug that is active in the body tissues and therefore able to exert a therapeutic effect.

brand name—The trademark under which individual manufacturers may market a drug.

broad-spectrum antibiotic—An antibiotic that is active against a wide range of bacteria.

bronchodilator—A drug that relaxes the bronchial muscles and expands the airways.

bronchospasm—Constriction of the muscles in the walls of the bronchioles.

bulk-forming laxatives—Fiber-containing products that promote the transit of stool by increasing stool bulk in order to distend the bowel. This, in turn, stimulates peristalsis (contraction of the bowels).

bursitis—Inflammation of a bursa.

calcium channel blocker—Antihypertensive medication that causes a reduction in calcium concentration in vascular smooth muscle cells, resulting in generalized vasodilation and subsequently decreasing systemic vascular resistance.

candidiasis—Any skin infection caused by the yeast *Candida*.

cephalosporins—A family of antibiotics that inhibit the synthesis of bacterial cell walls by attaching to specific enzymes responsible for cell wall construction. Closely related to the penicillins.

combination product—A product that contains two or more active ingredients. For example, many cough and cold remedies contain several active ingredients.

comparative negligence—The practice of assigning proportionate responsibility.

complex seizure—A partial seizure that involves an impairment of consciousness.

confidentiality—The respect you assign to the privacy of personal information provided to you by the athletes under your care.

contributory negligence—Fault on the part of the victim that contributed to an unexpected outcome.

controlled substances—Therapeutic drugs that may be sold on the street as potential drugs of abuse. The prescribing and sale of these drugs are controlled by the federal government.

corticosteroids—Steroid hormones produced within the adrenal cortex or synthetic versions of these hormones manufactured within a laboratory. Four types of corticosteroids are produced by the adrenal cortex: mineralocorticoids (aldosterone), glucocorticoids (cortisol), androgens, and estrogens.

counterirritant—An agent that causes irritation or mild inflammation of the skin with the objective of relieving pain.

COX-2—The cyclooxygenase enzyme believed to be primarily induced at sites of inflammation. This is the target enzyme of the "COX-2 selective" nonsteroidal anti-inflammatory drugs.

decongestants—Alpha-1 agonists that bind to the alpha-1 receptors on blood vessels in the nasal mucosa and cause vasoconstriction. This leads to a decrease in blood flow to the mucosa and a drying of secretions.

delayed-release tablets—A drug with a special coating that keeps the medication from dissolving in the stomach, or delays dissolution, and prolongs absorption of the tablet to lengthen the duration of effect.

depression—A condition that is characterized by clinically significant depression of mood and impairment of functioning. Symptoms of depression include persistent sad, anxious, or empty mood; feelings of hopelessness, pessimism, guilt, worthlessness, and helplessness; loss of interest or pleasure in hobbies and activities that were once enjoyed; fatigue and decreased energy; difficulty concentrating, remembering, and making decisions; insomnia, early-morning awakening, or oversleeping; and loss of appetite and weight loss or overeating and weight gain.

dermatophytid reaction—A secondary rash that appears separate from the actual site of the fungal infection. It is caused by an overreaction of the body's immune system.

diabetic ketoacidosis—A potentially fatal medical condition resulting from an increase in the amount of ketones in the body.

distribution—The process that allows a drug, once absorbed, to be spread by the circulatory system so that it can exert its intended therapeutic effects.

diuretic—Antihypertensive medication that decreases plasma volume by increasing urinary output.

elimination—The final process whereby the body removes a substance.

epilepsy—A disorder of brain function characterized by the periodic and unpredictable occurrence of seizures.

exercise-induced bronchospasm (EIB)—Asthmatic symptoms brought on by vigorous physical activity.

expectorant—A medication intended to thin mucus secretions of the respiratory tract and promote clearance by allowing a more productive cough.

floroquinolones—A family of antibiotics that exert their effect on bacteria by interfering with the coiling process of bacterial DNA.

Food and Drug Administration (FDA)—An agency of the U.S. Department of Health and Human Services that is responsible for overseeing the manufacture, labeling, and distribution of food, cosmetics, and other chemical substances, including therapeutic drugs.

food supplement—A substance that must contain at least one of the following: vitamins, minerals, herbs or botanicals, amino acids, metabolites, or constituents or extracts of any of these substances.

gastroesophageal reflux disease (GERD)—A condition that results from backward movement of gastric secretions from the stomach into the esophagus. Commonly referred to as *heartburn*.

generalized seizure—A seizure that arises from multiple parts of the brain.

generic name—The official, assigned name that a drug is licensed under by the FDA.

glucagon—A hormone produced by the alpha cells of the pancreas. Its role is to help the body maintain blood glucose levels.

glucocorticoid—A type of corticosteroid with multiple effects on the body's function; the primary effect is anti-inflammatory.

gluconeogenesis—The formation of glucose by the body from noncarbohydrate sources.

gram-negative bacteria—Organisms that absorb little or none of a specific dye and show up under a microscope as a faint pink color.

gram-positive bacteria—Organisms that absorb a specific dye and appear purple under microscopic magnification.

H2 receptor antagonists—Drugs that block the production of gastric acid. This is accomplished by inhibiting the release of histamine from parietal cells.

half-life—The time required for the body to eliminate one-half of a dosage of a drug by regular physical processes.

hydrocortisone—A commonly used topical corticosteroid.

hyperglycemia—Abnormally high blood glucose level.

hypersensitivity—An abnormal sensitivity that is likely to induce an overreaction to a specific substance.

hypoglycemia—Abnormally low blood glucose level.

infiltrative anesthesia—The injection of an anesthetic into the skin or around a nerve to achieve pain control and allow for suturing of a laceration, reduction of a fracture, or other potentially painful procedures.

influenza—A respiratory viral illness characterized by the abrupt onset of fever (100-104 °F; 38-40 °C), chills, cough, rhinorrhea, sore throat, malaise, myalgias, headache, and anorexia.

injectable anesthetics—Drugs such as lidocaine that can be injected into a joint or infiltrated into the skin to achieve anesthesia.

insulin—A hormone produced by the pancreas—or administered exogenously—that regulates the entry of glucose into cells.

isomers—Two molecules that have identical chemical compositions but are arranged differently, like left and right hands.

jock itch—A fungal infection (tinea cruris) that attacks the upper, inner thighs and groin area of men—especially those between the ages of 18 and 40—and is characterized by a red, scaly rash that is quite itchy.

lipid solubility—The ability of a drug to easily penetrate fat stores and cross cell membranes, including the blood-brain barrier.

macrolides—A family of antibiotics that inhibit bacterial protein synthesis. This class has a similar spectrum of activity to the penicillins and can be used in individuals with a penicillin allergy.

malpractice—Any actions taken that are outside a defined standard of care and that result in harm.

metabolism—A clearing process that is the sum of all chemical processes that take place in the body as they relate to the movement of nutrients in the blood, resulting in growth, energy, release of wastes, and other vital body functions.

MRSA—Methicillin-resistant *Staphylococcus aureus*. A bacterial strain that has been responsible for a number of outbreaks of cellulitis and boils across the country, both in hospitals and among athletic teams. It is resistant to a number of classes of antibiotics.

myoclonic seizure—Brief shocklike contractions of muscles restricted to one or more extremities.

narcotic—An addictive drug that reduces pain and also alters mood and behavior.

narrow-spectrum antibiotic—An antibiotic that is active against a specific type of bacteria.

non-anti-inflammatory agent—A drug (typically an analgesic) that is not a member of the NSAID family.

NSAID—A nonsteroidal anti-inflammatory drug.

opiate agonist—A drug that controls pain by stimulating specific opiate receptors throughout the body's central nervous system.

osmotic laxatives—Drugs that promote fluid retention in the colon by drawing fluid into the bowel.

over-the-counter (OTC) drugs—Legal medications available for purchase without a prescription.

partial seizure—A seizure that begins in one focal site of the brain.

peak serum concentration—The highest level of drug in the bloodstream following ingestion.

pediatric dose—Drugs for children are dosed according to age, weight, and body surface area.

penicillins—A family of antibiotics that inhibit the synthesis of bacterial cell walls by attaching to specific enzymes responsible for cell wall construction.

peptic ulcer disease (PUD)—A chronic inflammatory erosion of the GI tract mucosa, typically occurring in the stomach or duodenum.

pharmacodynamics—The study of the actions of drugs on living organisms.

pharmacokinetics—The study of how the body handles a drug.

pharmacology—The science of drugs, including their biochemistry, uses, and biological and therapeutic effects.

potency—An individual drug's strength.

proton pump inhibitors—Drugs that inhibit gastric acid production by blocking the release of hydrogen ions from gastric parietal cells.

receptor—A molecule within a cell or on the cell membrane that reacts with a drug and initiates a biological response that causes the drug to be therapeutic.

ringworm—A fungal infection (tinea corporis) characterized by skin eruptions that are scaly, itchy, red, and ring shaped.

seizure—A transient alteration of behavior caused by the disordered, synchronous, and rhythmic firing of populations of brain neurons.

shelf life—The time frame during which drugs remain effective for treating the condition they were developed to treat.

shingles—A painful rash caused by the same virus (herpes zoster) that causes chicken pox.

simple seizure—A partial seizure during which consciousness is preserved.

single-ingredient product—A product that contains only one active ingredient.

standard dose—The number of tablets to take per dose, how often to take the medication, and the maximum number of tablets the individual should ingest in a 24-hour period. This represents what researchers consider to be the safe, effective amount and the dosage frequency an individual needs to benefit from the drug.

standard of care—Those rules, actions, or conditions that have been defined to guide the practice of medicine, which investigators can use to evaluate the performance of caregivers.

steroid—A lipid-soluble hormone with a chemical structure similar to cholesterol. Many types of steroids are produced by the body.

street drugs—A term used to denote illicit substances—such as LSD, mescaline, heroin, and crack cocaine—that can be purchased for cash on the street.

tetanus—A potentially deadly infection of the central nervous system. It is caused by *Clostridium tetani* spores.

therapeutic drugs—Those substances that research has shown to have healing or curative powers.

tonic-clonic seizure—A seizure that involves a loss of consciousness and sustained contractions (tonic) of muscles throughout the body followed by periods of muscle contraction alternating with periods of relaxation (clonic).

topical analgesic—A drug that relieves pain when applied to the skin. This may be achieved through anesthesia or a counterirritant effect.

topical anesthetic—A drug that blocks nerve conduction and relieves pain when applied to the skin.

type 1 diabetes mellitus—A disease that results from the destruction of insulin-producing beta cells in the pancreas by an autoimmune process. Affected individuals typically require insulin administration to maintain normal blood sugar levels.

type 2 diabetes mellitus—A disease that results from a variety of factors, including diminished insulin production, problems with glucose production in the liver, and insulin resistance in peripheral tissues.

vasoconstrictor—A drug (such as epinephrine) that causes the constriction of blood vessels to control bleeding.

vasodilation—The dilation of blood vessels.

withdrawal syndrome—A condition that may result when the chronic use of opiate agonists is abruptly discontinued. Symptoms include fever, runny nose, sneezing, diarrhea, goose flesh, unusually large pupils, nervousness, irritability, and rapid heartbeat.

INDEX

Note: The letters *f* and *t* after page numbers indicate figures and tables, respectively.

ABOUT THE AUTHOR

Michael C. Koester, MD, ATC, FAAP, is a board-certified sports medicine specialist with over 20 years of experience in the evaluation and treatment of sports-related injuries and conditions. In addition to being a sports medicine physician, he is a certified athletic trainer and a member of the writing committee for NATA certification exams. He earned his BS in athletic training from the University of Nevada in 1992 and then went on to obtain his MD from University of Nevada School of Medicine in 1996. A sports medicine fellowship followed at Vanderbilt University, and he most recently became board certified in 2006. His areas of expertise in the active adult population are knee and shoulder injuries.